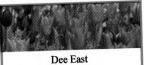
Love, Hono
& Value

A Family Caregiver Speaks Out
about the Choices and
Challenges of Caregiving

D0617610

Also by SUZANNE GEFFEN MINTZ

The Resourceful Caregiver:
Helping Family Caregivers Help Themselves

Love, Honor, & Value

A Family Caregiver Speaks Out about the Choices and Challenges of Caregiving

Suzanne Geffen Mintz

**President/Co-Founder,
National Family Caregivers Association**

Capital Books, Inc.
Sterling, Virginia

Capital Books, Inc.
P.O. Box 605
Herndon, Virginia 20172-0605

Library of Congress Cataloging-in-Publication Data

Mintz, Suzanne.
    Love, honor, & value / Suzanne Mintz.—1st ed.
        p. cm.
    Includes bibliographical references and index.
    ISBN 1-892123-56-8 (alk. paper)
    1. Caregivers.   2. Chronically ill—Care—Psychological aspects.   3. Care of the sick—Psychological aspects.   4. Stress management.   I. Title: Love, honor, and value   II. Title.
    RA645.35 .M54   2002
    362.1'01'9—dc21   2002023400

Printed in the United States of America on acid-free paper that meets the American National Standards Institute Z39-48 Standard.

First Edition

10 9 8 7 6 5 4 3 2 1

To Steven, Cindy, and Mom,
and in memory of Madeleine and Dad

Contents

Acknowledgments

This book could not have been written if family caregivers from around the country hadn't shared their thoughts, feelings, and ideas with me over the years. My first acknowledgment must go to them.

I am extremely grateful to my dear friends, Evie Rosen, Connie Ford Siskowski, and Alice Brauer—Evie for always reminding me to see my glass as at least half full, Connie for showing me the value of quiet persistence, and Alice for her ego-boosting and unwavering belief in my abilities.

A special thank you is owed to all of those individuals who in one way or another directly helped me with the preparation of this book.

It would have taken me so much longer to complete if Debra Weinreich hadn't sorted through all of the caregiver quotes that were e-mailed to me, organized them by relevant chapters, selected ones for possible use, and even suggested potential locations. I'm so pleased you bought the house next door and have become my friend.

Thanks to Deborah Halpern, Kris Kohlman, John Paul Marosy, and Nancy Miller for reading the draft of the book and giving me your honest comments. The book is so much better for your efforts.

Thanks to all of NFCA's Caregiver Community Action Network Volunteers, too numerous to mention, who were patient with my many e-mails regarding the book's title.

And thanks to Jeannie Ervin for sending out e-mails to so many family caregivers and printing out the hundreds of responses that all the great quotes have been drawn from, and to the rest of the NFCA staff, Margaret Fowles and Christal

Willingham. Thank you all so much for what you've done to support me in this effort, especially during the spring of 2001.

Thanks to Gary Barg for putting me in touch with Kathleen Hughes. Thanks to Kathleen for believing I could write this book, and thanks to Ann Santos who many years ago gave me the opportunity to write a column for PN.

Thanks to Cindy for being such a big part of my life for so many years, for helping to birth and grow NFCA, and for always being there when I've needed you.

And to Steven for putting up with so much, for allowing me to tell our story, and for being my inspiration and my strength.

All proceeds due the author
from the sale of *Love, Honor, & Value*
are being donated to the
National Family Caregivers Association.
NFCA is a 501(c)3 Organization.
Tax ID # is 52-1780405

Foreword

I first met Suzanne Mintz at a conference on caregiving and long-term care. I'd heard that she was a passionate caregiver with a good grasp of the issues and a vision of how caregiving families should be treated. After meeting her, I knew why. Bound by the zeal that only a person with first-hand experience as a caregiver can bring, Suzanne has become an advocate extraordinaire for caregiving families. Putting in words the thoughts and feelings of millions of family caregivers, she gives a voice to the voiceless and minimizes the frustration that so often comes to those who provide care for a chronically ill, disabled, or aged loved one.

Launching a national organization, the National Family Caregivers Association (NFCA), was the logical step when she and long-time friend Cindy Fowler realized that family caregiving is a lifespan issue that brings similar concerns and problems regardless of relationship or a loved one's diagnosis. Today NFCA is the largest and most influential organization for family caregivers in the country, providing information and education, support and validation, and public awareness and advocacy, all in an effort to make life better for family caregivers and their loved ones. And now this book, which provides personal accounts, hers and many others, combined with practical advice and a call to action for family caregivers, is here to make sure their voices are heard, and their difficulties are known to other family members and friends, within their local communities, and in the halls of county, state, and national government.

Family Caregiver Alliance (FCA), the San Francisco-based organization I am proud to direct, was created out of similar circumstances. Individual family caregivers Anne Bashkiroff and Suzanne Harris were willing to talk about their private experiences in public so others would not have to face the isolation, confusion, and lack of support from the medical community created by their role as primary providers of care for their loved ones with Alzheimer's. Their efforts and those of a few other caregiver advocates and interested professionals gave birth to what is now a twenty-five-year-old organization known nationwide for its ability to provide policy makers, program developers, and researchers with the information they need to further their work in assisting family caregivers.

It's hard to believe that from such humble beginnings as these, from the fire of a few, so much can happen. And yet that is the way of progress and change, and NFCA and FCA have proved that a few committed people really can make a difference. Many other grassroots organizations can trace their history back to a few advocates who defined a dream and enlisted the support of others to make it come true. Advocates tell their stories in an effort to right the wrongs they see and experience on a daily level, and in the process heighten the awareness and bring forth the hidden energy of others. They plant the seeds of a movement they may never have imagined possible.

Caregiving families face innumerable challenges on a daily basis. Changes in the care a loved one needs means getting used to a whole new reality. Some caregivers learn to anticipate. Others can't and are always thrown into crisis. Family and friends drift away after the acute stage of an illness is over because they are uncomfortable facing the reality of growing disability or unusual behaviors. Simultaneous work and care responsibilities squeeze all personal time from the calendar of caregivers. Denying their own health problems in the face of daily caregiving demands unfortunately is commonplace. All of these experiences are part of the reality of being a family caregiver, and they all come to life in this book through the quotes of caregivers from across the country.

"At each step we have tried to anticipate the next problem dad would be facing. . . . This forward thinking has helped us not have to scramble and has helped us be mentally prepared as changes occurred."

Indiana

"A lot of people don't want to be around someone who is sick. Some friends may never call or stop by again."

California

"After three months I had lost twenty pounds, had terrible bags under my eyes, and looked like a zombie. The doctor threatened to hospitalize me because I was suffering from exhaustion."

New Jersey

These conditions pose problems for family caregivers. Although they are lived out in individual lives, they demand service solutions that are comprehensive in approach, solutions that acknowledge all caregivers' rights to information, sources of support, recognition of their own physical and mental health issues, and legal and financial considerations.

Family caregivers really are the "care coordinators" of their family. Long-term care is not measured in months or by individual crises, but rather by years and maintenance of function for loved ones. Family caregivers are the historians and managers of their loved one's medical, social, financial, and cultural lives. Seen in this light, it is clear that the issues involved in supporting family caregivers are complex. They are personal. They are familial. And yes, they are societal, too. Yet, so many family caregivers are unaware that all of these issues are swirling around them and that more than 50 million other Americans just like them are providing some level of care to a loved one in need. The isolation that so often accompanies caregiving deprives them of even the slim support that knowing they are not alone can provide.

Love, Honor, & Value explores what this means in the everyday lives of family caregivers, and what each of us might be able to do to meet our individual challenges. It discusses why caregiving is different today than it ever was in the past, and suggests what society ought to do to integrate family caregiving into the fabric of our healthcare system. It honors the work of family caregivers by explaining how caregivers are actually members of their loved one's healthcare team, and how much knowledge of their loved one's condition they bring to the table.

By combining the story of her personal journey with a call to action, Suzanne has made a difference in the lives of the family caregivers who have heard her speak or who have read her articles. Now, with the publication of this book, many more people will have the chance to learn, to feel, to be inspired, and in some cases to follow her lead.

Thanks, Suzanne, for coming forward with your story so others may not have to face the isolation, confusion, and lack of support so common with families caring for their loved ones. And thank you for starting the National Family Caregivers Association so that caregivers all across the country, regardless of their circumstances, can know there is a better way and that there are many of us around the country working to make a vision of a better world for caregiving families come true.

Kathleen A. Kelly
Executive Director
Family Caregiver Alliance

Introduction

Marjorie is a family caregiver, a person who provides essential, unpaid assistance to a relative or friend who is ill, elderly, or disabled. The two parts of the term are equally important. "Family" denotes a special personal relationship with the care recipient; one based on birth, adoption, marriage, or declared commitment. "Caregiver" is the job description, which may include providing personal care, carrying out medical procedures, managing a household, and interacting with the formal health-care and social service systems on another's behalf. Caregivers are more than the sum of their responsibilities; they are real people with complex and often conflicted responses to the situations they face.

This is the best description of a family caregiver that I have ever read. It was written by Carol Levine, Director of the Families and Health Care Project at the United Hospital Fund of New York. It appears in a book she edited titled *Always on Call When Illness Turns Families into Caregivers*. It has the mark of her professional knowledge about caregiving issues in our time, and her very personal understanding of what it means to be a family caregiver for more than a dozen years beginning when her husband was severely injured in an automobile accident.

Carol's distinction between the word *family* as the definer of a caring relationship and the word *caregiver* as the description of a job is an important one. Putting the two together as a single term is what distinguishes you and me from others who provide care, such as doctors, nurses, home care aides, and members of the clergy, none of whom fit the description above, largely because the care they provide stems from the

xvi   **Love, Honor, and Value**

professions they have chosen to pursue. Nonetheless, these professionals think of themselves as caregivers and so does the wider world.

This book is about family caregivers, not professional ones. It uses the term *family caregiver* in the broadest sense possible and it uses the term *family caregiver* and the word *caregiver* interchangeably. It was written primarily for family members, friends, and partners giving care, including those who are just beginning a caregiving journey, those for whom family caregiving is an integral part of their daily lives, and also those who aren't even sure if what they are doing is really family caregiving at all. Although it speaks directly to family caregivers, I hope it will also find a ready audience among members of the health and social services communities whose work puts them in direct contact with family caregivers. I hope care recipients, family, and friends will pick it up and find value in these pages, as well.

It has been difficult for me to define the exact nature of this book. It isn't a caregiver's memoir, although it certainly contains personal information about my own caregiving experience. It's not the explanation of a philosophy, although it does propose a way to cope with life as a family caregiver. It's not a workbook, although it does ask questions and provide suggestions for activities. And it is not a collection of other caregiver's thoughts, feelings, and ideas, although these are definitely sprinkled throughout the book.

I invite you to read it and decide for yourself. My intent has been to bring solace, hope, and potentially some new ways of looking at life to those of you who are currently family caregivers, and some insights and ideas to make your journey easier if you anticipate becoming a family caregiver in the future. If you are a care receiver, a relative, friend, healthcare or social services professional, or member of the clergy, I hope it will give you a deeper understanding of the complexities of what it means to love and care for someone who is chronically ill, disabled, or aged.

I've written the book based on the information, and, I hope, the wisdom, I have gained from my own ongoing caregiving journey, and the knowledge, empathy, and education I have gained since co-founding the National Family Caregivers Association (NFCA) almost ten years ago. It is my sincere hope that what I have to share with you will make a positive difference in your life, your loved one's life, and the lives of at least some of the millions of other Americans who are trying to find their way through the maze of caregiving in our fractured and "quicker and sicker" healthcare system.

Suzanne Mintz
Kensington, MD
January 2002

CHAPTER 1

In Sickness
and in Health

It all began on a Sunday afternoon in the fall of 1974 when my husband Steven started feeling a tingling sensation in both legs. He tried shaking them, the way you do when they've "fallen sleep," but that didn't make the tingling sensation go away. It persisted during the rest of the day and throughout the night. So, in the morning, Steven called our internist and friend, Dr. Hal Mirsky, in the hope of getting an appointment later that day. Hal advised otherwise. "I think you should see a neurologist rather than me," he said. "I'll give you a referral." That's how we met Dr. Richard Edelson. After hearing a description of Steven's symptoms and doing a number of non-invasive tests in his office, Dr. Edelson said that Steven should enter George Washington University Hospital right away. More tests were necessary. It was obvious that something was definitely wrong, and both Steven and I started to get scared.

He was in the hospital for four or five days. It's hard to remember exactly. Time didn't seem to be following its regular steady pattern then. Some days a second felt like an hour, and on other days hours flew by like seconds as I tried to keep up with the normal routine of life and spend as much time at the hospital with Steven as was possible.

Some of the tests didn't seem like tests at all. The doctor

would bang Steven's knees with a triangular shaped hammer to see how quickly they jutted forward. He asked him lots of questions. "Do you ever recall not being able to get one of your legs to respond in the normal way, either while you were walking or running? Do you ever recall stubbing your toe while climbing stairs? Any problems seeing? Any difficulty picking up things with your hands? Do you get overly fatigued in the heat?" The questions horrified me, one of Steven's answers even more. He acknowledged having a problem with his right leg from time to time. That explained, to me at least, why he always had an excuse for not wanting to play basketball with the other men in our garden apartment complex. An athlete and sports lover, he wasn't willing to join the game if he couldn't perform at the level he was used to. But there was some good news coupled with the bad. The problem, whatever it was, seemed to be localized. Symptoms had never appeared anywhere other than in his right leg.

Dr. Edelson ordered a number of tests that in themselves were frightening. For one of them, a mylogram, Steven was strapped to a table and turned upside down. A dye was injected into his spinal column so that the doctors could watch the dye on a monitor as it flowed from the base of his spinal column all the way up into his neck. They wanted to see if there were any blockages along the column that might explain the tingling. The test was done while Steven was wide awake because it was vital that he be conscious and not move even a fraction of an inch so that the dye wouldn't flow further than intended. If the dye entered his brain there might well have been brain damage. He still recalls his anxiety and fear as he watched the dye flow ever closer to his brain and the point of danger and the sigh of relief he let out when the test was finally over.

Another test would give him significant headaches, he was warned. It involved inserting a needle into his spinal column and drawing out fluid. The fluid would then be tested to measure the level of various proteins, especially gamma globulin.

Although it wouldn't prove anything conclusively, we were told, given the technology of the time it was our best shot at finding out what was wrong. He should expect the headaches to last about two weeks, until his body had time to regenerate the lost spinal fluid and restore its balance. Although the test was dangerous—removing spinal fluid is not an inconsequential act—we decided Steven should go ahead with it. We wanted to know what was happening to his body and why.

Some images from that time are still very vivid for me. I recall the evenings when Steven was in the hospital. After our daughter Darryn, all of five years old, had been put to bed, and I finished my chores and homework (I was in graduate school at the time), I'd get into bed myself, emotionally and physically weary, and I would cry. Violent sobs would escape from my mouth, and I would try to muffle them with my hand, afraid that Darryn might wake and want to know why I was crying. I'd lie there, arms crossed in front of my chest, squeezing my upper arms, trying without much success to feel that I was being held and comforted. "Perhaps he'll need an operation, perhaps he'll need an operation, perhaps he'll need an operation," I said silently to myself, seeing brain surgery not as something to fear but rather the potential answer to my prayers. I prayed to God, who I never before believed was a direct interventionist in our individual lives, but who during those nights I fervently wished was. I prayed that Steven would be well. I wanted to know what was happening to his body. I wanted an answer. I wanted whatever was wrong to be made right. Eventually I would fall asleep and wake in the morning as tired as I had been when I went to bed.

There are some memories from that time that are more than vivid. They are imprinted on my heart forever. The moment I heard Steven's diagnosis is one of them. The details are still crystal clear, even though it happened more than twenty-five years ago.

It was a crisp, sunny day in October. I had gone to the hospital, and as I was getting off the elevator the attending physician on duty came over to me. "I was hoping I would see you," he said, guiding me to the waiting area, a rather public and very uninviting space furnished with cheap plastic molded chairs that were lined up in rows facing each other.

"Your husband has multiple sclerosis," he continued, without emotion. "MS is a degenerative and incurable neurological disease. I'm sorry." An image from childhood flashed through my mind, the image of a neighbor who had MS. I would see her, on sunny days, sitting on her front porch in a wheelchair, as I walked up the street with the jaunty step of a preteen on the way to play with a friend. I don't recall if I ever said hello. I hope I did. I now envisioned Steven in a wheelchair, wrapped up in a blanket the way Mrs. Schmirer always was, waiting for someone to bring him a glass of water with a straw, or wheel him back into the house. It was so terrifying it took my breath away. I was twenty-eight years old when Steven was diagnosed with MS. He was thirty-one. From that moment on, our lives and Darryn's were irrevocably changed.

Steven had a very different reaction to the news. He didn't know anything about MS. He'd never seen anyone with it. No images popped into his head. The words didn't create the same sense of fear and dread in him that they immediately did in me. The doctor had told him the same things he had told me and so he was scared about what could happen—who wouldn't be—but no specific images, no memories of real people haunted him.

Not long after he was diagnosed I heard that people with multiple sclerosis have a high divorce rate. Whether it is true or not I don't really know. I never actually wanted to find out for fear that it would happen to us. It wouldn't surprise me though. The vagaries of the disease, its often on-again-off-again nature, its degenerative path, and the fact that it usually attacks just when a person is spreading his or her adult wings, all conspire to eat away at the tender core of a marriage. MS has no specific prognosis, no timetable, no cure. If it's mild, symptoms may recede or go away entirely for long periods of time. If it's more virulent, the damage accumulates in very visible ways. Today there are drugs that help slow the progress of the disease, but in 1974 there wasn't anything of the sort available. Flare-ups could be treated, but the disease would take its own willful course. That's one of the things that makes it so devastating. There's nothing about MS you can hang your hat on, nothing that points the way to a specific plan of action. You know it's there. The words have been uttered. It is now part of your medical history. Like an uninvited guest that has made himself at home, it has somehow become a permanent part of your family.

When Steven came home from the hospital, the tingles had stopped, and nothing seemed different about him. He'd stub a toe on a step now and then, unable to move his foot in quite the right way to climb easily from riser to riser, but that was all. Why make anyone worry, we thought, deciding not to tell our parents, all four of whom lived in Florida, or even our closest friends who we saw all the time and thought of as family. But I desperately needed to feel I wasn't on my own in dealing with the knowledge of Steven's diagnosis and my fears about our future. So we took Steven's sister and brother-in-law into our confidence. It helped a little, but the fact that they too lived far away meant I still didn't have a shoulder to cry on in the literal sense.

Outwardly, the pattern of our lives didn't change. Darryn entered first grade. I completed my master's degree and got a part-time job with a design firm—my first paid employment since she was born—and Steven continued to work as an economist for the federal government.

Everything seemed normal, but nothing was. Our sensitivities were so heightened that the simplest question. "How was your day?" took on a new significance. The response, "It was tiring," conjured up an invalid's lifestyle. I was apprehensive, unsure of what might happen from day to day, unsure of every conversation, unsure of being too solicitous or of not showing enough concern. Steven's health became a major topic of conversation. It consumed our attention and stifled me, but I couldn't admit it. I couldn't say, "Let's not talk about how you feel all of the time. Let's try and live as normal a life as possible."

Steven, never one to share much about his inner feelings, shared even less of them then. I didn't know whether he felt the same about the turn our conversations had taken. I didn't know what he needed to quiet his personal fear of the unknown, but I later learned neither did he. We were hurting very badly, grieving the loss of what we thought life should and would be like. Neither one of us had any immediate answers. We were both just trying, in our different ways, to survive emotionally.

On top of the confusion and pain that Steven's diagnosis brought into our lives, another catastrophic event occurred nine months later. This one happened to me, to my body. I was raped. At home. In my own bed. Steven was away on a business trip. Darryn was asleep in the next room and a man broke into our apartment. He woke me out of a deep sleep, pulled the blanket over my head, and said, "If you don't stay quiet and keep your eyes covered, I'll bruise you." Once I became fully conscious and realized what was happening, my greatest fear was that Darryn would wake up and walk into my bedroom. What might happen then? What would he do to her? I lay there as he commanded, not moving a muscle, and when he got what he came for, he left as silently as he had come. It happened relatively quickly and without any violence whatsoever. It would have been easy to think I had imagined it, but I knew I hadn't, and so with the day slowly dawning outside my window, I called 911.

The police who came in response to my call, a man and a woman, were great. They treated me with respect and compassion. They said I'd have to go to the hospital and have an internal examination to corroborate my story. For the second time in the space of only a few hours I was to have a stranger explore the most intimate part of my body. A neighbor took Darryn, and off I went in the police car. Once at the hospital I remember sitting on the examination table waiting and waiting and waiting for the doctor to appear. The policewoman stayed with me the whole time. I was so grateful. A social worker came in and gave me her card. "Call me," she said. "I think it will be good for you to talk about this." Finally the doctor came, unceremoniously examined me, and said that, yes, I had definitely been raped. Then he left and I was free to go home. I had no physical wounds that needed to heal, so there were no outward physical reminders of my ordeal, but for months I heard the rapist's voice in my ears, and I wonder to this very day if the emotional wounds he left behind have fully healed, or if they ever will.

The police never did find out who the rapist was, nor how he got into our apartment. The balcony faced dark woods, and they thought he might have climbed up the railing to our third-floor apartment and entered through the sliding glass doors. We also never found out if it was a random act or if I was the intended victim. With all that uncertainty, neither Steven nor I felt safe in the apartment, and for Steven, it was a constant reminder that he hadn't been home that night, even though he knew that if he had been, the outcome might have been worse than it was.

The bad memories and unanswered questions prompted us to buy our first house, a happy event brought about by unhappy circumstances. We bought a ranch-style house, just in case Steven wouldn't be able to climb stairs one day. The change of scene was helpful, but in the months and years that followed Steven and I were overwhelmed with what had happened to each of our bodies and to our collective life.

We needed to come to terms with the two great losses we

had suffered, and we didn't know how. We each needed to grieve, but didn't understand why, or know that grieving is a very personal act that each of us needs to experience in our own way, according to our inner workings. Little did we know that our two grieving styles and coping mechanisms were completely opposite. Little did we know that our inability to share what we were each really thinking and feeling and needing would soon have a disastrous effect on our relationship.

Steven's natural inclination is to turn inward for strength. I need to reach out for support. It never occurred to us that these differences would cause us to end up waging an emotional war against one another, a war that would lead to a ten-month separation, followed by an eighteen-month truce and another separation, this one lasting two full years, before we finally realized just how different we were emotionally. It was a profound awakening when we came to understand that neither Steven's way of coping nor mine was better, but rather that our differences needed to be recognized and respected if we were to live comfortably together under one roof again. The understanding came in a flash—all of a sudden it was there—but lots of talking and, at least for me, lots of counseling preceded it.

Darryn lived with me during the two years we were apart, but she saw Steven every weekend and helped him with the groceries. We were constantly concerned about her reaction to Steven's increasing disability and our separation. Her best friend's dad was disabled, and her parents were divorced, so the girls became an emotional lifeline for each other and developed a very deep bond that continues to this day. Darryn constantly assured me that she was okay, and I had no reason not to take her at her word, but I was also glad that she had Shannon to talk to during those difficult times.

Like most couples, Steven and I had married "for better or for worse, in sickness and in health." But nobody who marries at twenty-one, as I did, or at twenty-three as was the case with Steven, thinks that means anything more serious than the common cold. No young couple expects tragedy to invade their lives.

I think the reason we were able to heal our marriage despite the many serious injuries it had received is that underneath it all we really are quite good for each other. Darryn said it best, when we asked her if she had been concerned that we might actually get divorced. "No," she responded. "I knew you guys loved each other." So after years of turmoil and heartache, we got together again, this time truly for better or for worse, but the hardest part was still ahead.

Steven has the slow continually degenerating variety of MS, technically called "primary progressive." It is the least common of the three types. Like a leaky faucet that only attracts attention after water starts to collect visibly in the basin, primary progressive MS drips into your life. By 1979, five years after his diagnosis, Steven's basin was filling up. His gait was uneven, his balance a bit off. We couldn't hide it anymore. We told our parents and friends. We told Darryn. Two years later he started to use a cane. Toward the end of 1982 he got a pair of crutches, the kind with arm supports for more stability.

Then early in 1985, about ten years after he was diagnosed, Steven bought a motorized scooter to get around at work, in shopping malls, and other places where lots of walking was required. The scooter was a great relief to me. I no longer had to watch him struggle to walk a block. I no longer had to worry if he was going to fall and break his neck. The scooter gave us back some long lost freedom. It made it easier to go places—as long as they were accessible. On the other hand, the scooter was a reminder that the MS was here to stay, an unwanted, permanent lodger in our home.

After numerous conversations with myself over the years, I had set a timetable for Steven's increasing disability that I thought I could live with. I accepted the possibility, even the probability, that he might end up in a wheelchair in his mid fifties. When he needed the wheelchair thirteen years ahead of "my schedule," extreme sadness mixed with a lot of hidden anger overtook me. As Steven became more and more disabled, I became a classic example of Freudian sublimation. I couldn't admit my pain or my anger, so I channeled most of my energy into work-related activities instead. I concentrated on my career and was always so busy between work, being a mom, and being a homemaker, that I literally didn't have time to dwell on Steven's worsening physical condition.

But pushing myself didn't make the pain go away. It didn't resolve my grief. Instead it turned anger into anguish and then into clinical depression that required a long period of intensive therapy and medication before it ended, before I regained my mental and emotional equilibrium. For the first time since Steven had come home from the hospital those many years before, I let myself cry and through my tears began to heal.

If you've never suffered from depression, or even spent time with someone who has, it is a very difficult disease to comprehend. The chemical imbalance that occurs in the brain during periods of clinical depression somehow causes feelings of dread, fear, and anxiety to take over. For me, depression appears as a dark menacing cloud directly over my head, even on a sunny day. The cloud is ominous and jagged, not fluffy and white. It bears down on me as if it were a heavy steel plate and makes it hard for me stand up straight. The pain is unbearable, although it isn't a physical pain. All I want is for it to stop because life seems worthless if it won't go away. The pressure of the cloud on my head and back causes me to lose all my self-confidence. Making decisions, even very simple ones, such as whether to buy white bread or whole wheat, becomes unbearably difficult, and thus another source of pain and anguish. I lose my appetite during bouts of depression and can't sleep more than an hour or two at a time. The irony of it all is that all I seem to want to do during those times is get into bed and pull the covers over my head so I won't have to face the world, so I won't have to feel.

These bouts of depression, which began in 1986 and have come and gone three times since, are terrible for Steven. He feels helpless in his wheelchair with his limited dexterity. But I tell him he is my lifeline, and if I didn't need to physically assist him every day, I might never make the effort to care for myself. I tell him that even though he can't really do anything for me physically, he gives me the emotional strength to fight the depression. At times like this I know how important it is to have someone who loves you close by. That is one of the key factors for me in getting well, but I also know I can't do it without medication and talk therapy, both of which help restore me to health. The medication works on the chemicals in my brain that are out of whack, and the talk therapy gives me the opportunity, the permission, to confront my demons and better understand them.

William Styron, the Pulitzer prize winning writer perhaps best known as the author of *Sophie's Choice* and *The Confessions of Nat Turner*, has suffered from depression. He wrote about his experience in the book *Darkness Visible: A Memoir of Madness*.

What I had begun to discover is that, mysteriously and in ways that are totally remote from normal experience, the gray drizzle of horror induced by depression takes on the quality of physical pain. But it is not an immediately identifiable pain, like that of a broken limb. It may be more accurate to say that despair, owing to some evil trick played upon the sick brain by the inhabiting psyche, comes to resemble the diabolical discomfort of being imprisoned in a fiercely overheated room. And because no breeze stirs this caldron, because there is no escape from this smothering confinement, it is entirely natural that the victim begins to think ceaselessly of oblivion.

After Steven read the book he told me that although he had lived through periods of depression with me and saw it first hand, the book gave him an appreciation for what I was going through that he hadn't had before, that he could not have imagined. Try as I might, I don't have a similar appreciation for the extreme and enervating fatigue that sometimes overtakes him without warning, or the anguish that causes him to scream in frustration when he tries to slide his feet just one inch along the bathroom floor, and no matter how hard he tries they stay solidly rooted to the tile. I imagine the exhaustion. I see the struggle, but I know they are nothing compared to his reality.

There's a subtle difference between giving in, hanging on, and graciously accepting the inevitable. Steven and I had to learn to deal with these various perspectives. We had to recognize that we tend to do these things in very different ways. What we learned is that we needed to find a way to satisfy both of our competing grieving and coping styles. What ultimately got us back together, and has kept us together, was the recognition that although he is the one with clinical MS, "We," the family Mintz, also have MS, at least in a psycho-social sense. Steven's needs must be met, but so must mine.

Steven's a quiet fighter. He stretches his ability to the limit, grabbing for each piece of independence he can preserve. Not wanting to let the MS get the upper hand, he will struggle to maintain his current level of activity as long as possible. Even when he might have easily fallen down the stairs, when it was clearly beyond his ability to continue climbing or descending them safely, he would keep on, even if it took him a half hour or forty-five minutes, rather than admit defeat. I admire that greatly, but I ached inside each time I watched him struggle to do what most of us can do so easily. I didn't always admire this quality in him. In fact I used to hate it because I thought he was just being stubborn, and sometimes even mean. I didn't appreciate that like Don Quixote, fighting the invisible foe is what he needs to do in order to survive emotionally.

Steven and I have learned, the hard way, that understanding

and accepting each other's inner needs, knowing each other's devils, is a great deal harder than understanding and accepting more obvious ones. But when we do, we have a treasure to last a lifetime.

Despite the fact that he now needs help with the standard "activities of daily living"—dressing, bathing, toileting, eating, mobility, and transferring—our lives are good for the time being. We share the things we always have—going to the movies and the theatre, reading mysteries, doing crossword puzzles, listening to jazz, and eating good food. We miss dancing and "standing-up hugs," the latter probably more than anything, but we are grateful that Steven is still working, and fulltime at that. Three days a week he uses a specially modified minivan with a built-in ramp, hand controls, and a locking system that safely allows him to drive from his wheelchair to the headquarters of the Department of Energy in Washington, D.C. The other two days he telecommutes by computer from our home. (Thank heaven for modern technology.) Darryn is all grown up. She's married and has made us grandparents, which is as great an experience as everyone always says it is.

I don't know what sort of a person I would have turned into without the tragedies that befell Steven and me, but I do know that I have done things and have an approach to life now that I never could have imagined if our lives had been easier. I am glad for my added character, my achievements, my compassion, but I would trade all of it in a heartbeat if it meant that I could wake up one morning and Steven was well.

CHAPTER 2

The Common Bonds of Caregiving

On a bright and sunny weekend in September of 1991, after school had reopened and the crush of vacationers had left the beach, but while the weather was still delightfully warm, I went away for the weekend with my long-time friend Cindy Fowler. We went for a respite from the pressure of our lives.

Cindy was caring for her seventy-eight-year-old mother, Madeleine, who was suffering from Parkinson's disease. Madeleine had moved from Kansas City and lived somewhat independently in the small apartment above the Fowler's garage at that time, but soon afterward moved into the spare bedroom in the Fowler's house. Madeleine had been living with Cindy, her husband Rich, their thirteen-year-old son Chris, and their foster son Huong for three years when Cindy and I went off for our weekend fling.

I had been dealing with Steven's illness for seventeen years, and he had severe mobility problems by then. He'd been using a scooter for years to get around out of doors, but moving around in the house had also become difficult and dangerous and now he was using a wheelchair at home. He could still get in and out of bed himself, dress himself, and take care of his other personal needs, albeit slowly and by holding on to walls and counter tops in the process. For all intents and purposes you could say he was able to function independently inside the house. The fact that his disability was, and is to this day, only physical meant I knew he could make wise decisions should something out of the ordinary occur. Under those circumstances I could go away for the weekend without worrying a great deal and without needing to make elaborate arrangements for his care.

And so we went, leaving after work on a Friday evening and looking forward to a pleasant three-and-a-half-hour drive to Dewey Beach, Delaware and the beach house of a friend who had graciously lent it to me for the weekend. But about an hour into the drive we hit stop-and-go traffic that soon turned into a complete standstill because of what we later learned was a very serious accident up ahead, an accident so serious that it required Medivac helicopters to transport injured people to a trauma center in Baltimore.

As night came on and we were sitting in the dark closed environment of the car, we began to talk to each other in a way we never had before. Cindy was a very private person at that time in her life. I didn't often know much about her inner thoughts, her hidden worries, but that night in the intimacy of the car she opened up and began talking about her concerns regarding Madeleine, about the difficulty of getting helpful information, about the emotional and growing physical impact caring for her mom was having on her. She knew my story fairly well. She had seen Steven deteriorating over the years, and in fact she and her husband Rich were the first friends Steven publicly told that he had MS. She knew the emotional pressures that the MS had caused in our lives, about our separations, and about my early bouts with depression. But despite this we had never talked about our fears, asked each other practical questions about providing care, or recognized that there were similarities in our situation. That night we did.

It was as if the proverbial light bulb went on, and it stayed on that entire weekend. As we sat on the beach and soaked up the sun, as we sat on the screened porch of the house after dinner and sipped a cup of coffee, and as we drove home in the light of day on Sunday afternoon, we talked, asked each other questions, discussed our concerns about the future, and realized that, although Cindy was caring for her mom and I was assisting my husband, that although Madeleine was elderly and had Parkinson's disease and Steven was still in his forties and had MS, we were feeling the same anguish, the same emotional distress and were concerned about similar issues. And we wondered why it seemed that no one recognized these similarities. We wondered why no one seemed to be focused on the fact that helping a loved one with a deteriorating illness had a very real impact on not only the person with the illness, but also on those of us who were primarily responsible for helping them.

We somehow knew the term *family caregiver*, although neither of us could say when we had first heard it. But know it we did, and now recognized that despite the differences between our circumstances, it applied to us equally. We were family caregivers, not solely that of course, but caregiving was a very real part of who we were, and we wanted people to take notice. We were family caregivers, and we wanted someone to reach out to us, to tell us where to find helpful information and advice, emotional support, and real hands-on assistance when we needed it. We weren't looking for, nor did we want, a pat on the back because we were caring for a family member we dearly loved, but we did want recognition of the difficulties involved. We wanted these things, but as far as we knew they didn't exist, or if they did, they weren't readily available.

We had been good friends before, but now we recognized this common bond. We now instinctively knew that we were not alone, that there must be thousands more people like us, thousands more family caregivers, needing what we needed, sharing common concerns, feeling the same emotions, needing much of the same kind of help and information. That spark of recognition was what ignited our desire to "do something," but do what, we did not know.

Cindy is a graphic designer and the president of her own award-winning design firm, Graves Fowler Associates. At the time, I was the principal in charge of marketing for a leading interior architectural firm in Washington, D.C. Cindy knew how to design a newsletter. I was itching to do some writing separate and apart from what I did as part of my job. At some point during the ride home from the beach the idea to try and create a newsletter for family caregivers was hatched, a newsletter that spoke to the common needs and concerns of family caregivers, regardless of whether they were caring for a spouse, or a parent, or a child, or a sibling, and regardless of what disease or disability their loved one had.

We didn't have a grand plan, just pent up emotion, an idea, and a desire to make a difference. And thus we began. I wrote the articles. Cindy did the design, and through her professional connections we were able to have the first newsletter, all four pages of it, printed for free. We called the newsletter *TAKE CARE! Self Care for the Family Caregiver,* and thus began our journey.

We made contact with the social work departments of local hospitals, met with a number of voluntary health agencies (that's the official name for groups such as the Alzheimer's Association, the National Multiple Sclerosis Society, and the American Cancer Society). We showed them the newsletter and asked them to share it with others. We requested individuals to give us five dollars if they wanted to receive future issues by mail.

A respite weekend at the beach. Two friends share the intimacy of time away together. Thoughts and feelings are expressed, an idea is born, and a toe is put into the water of the lake of good intentions to test the temperature of commitment and capabilities. Our temperature must have been right on because, two years later in the spring of 1993, *TAKE CARE!* became the official publication of the new organization we had formed: National Family Caregivers Association (NFCA).

Much has happened since those tentative days. NFCA has grown and changed. Today it is the nation's leading grassroots caregiver constituency organization, and the only one that reaches across the life span and the boundaries of differing diagnoses and relationships to address the common issues of all family caregivers. NFCA was created to educate, support, empower, and speak up for America's family caregivers so that all caregiving families can have a better quality of life. If you would like to find out more about NFCA, visit our web site: www.nfcacares.org.

The Weaver's Thread

What is the common thread that caregiving weaves through our lives, that Cindy and I discovered during our wonderful respite weekend at the beach? What is the single thread that ties together those of us who care for spouses, children, parents, siblings, partners, or friends who are chronically ill, frail, or disabled?

The common thread certainly isn't the tasks of caregiving. They vary so much, from helping a developmentally delayed child learn new skills, to taking an aging parent to frequent doctor's appointments, or suctioning a spinal chord injured spouse virtually every hour every day. The tasks of caregiving can differ tremendously from situation to situation.

It surely isn't the number of years involved. Caregiving can last a few short months, as when you are caring for a terminal cancer patient. It can last three to five years when caring for an aged parent who has a weak heart. At times, caregiving can be a lifetime commitment for a family, especially when a severely disabled child is involved.

Location varies from situation to situation. Although the

vast majority of caregiving goes on in the home and many caregivers and recipients live under the same roof, talk to anyone whose parent is in a nursing home, or whose child lives in a group home, and you'll quickly learn that caregiving doesn't end when someone else is responsible for day-to-day care, or when caregiving takes place long distance. Different situations have different demands and require different capabilities and commitments from us.

If it isn't the responsibilities or tasks, and it isn't the length of time, if it isn't the location, what is the essential bond that knits all family caregivers together? What does caring for a spouse with heart disease have to do with caring for parents who are losing their ability to live independently, or a child with spina bifida?

If you read caregivers' letters, if you listen to their stories as I have, it is very clear that the thread woven through the lives of all caregivers is the emotional impact of caregiving. Listen to these statements. Can you tell whether they were written by a spouse, or a parent, a partner, a loving friend, a sibling, an adult child or grandchild, or someone in another caregiving relationship? Can you tell which disease or disability their loved one has?

> *I feel overwhelmed most of the time and accomplish very little except meeting our immediate needs.*

> *I have nurses during the day to care for _____ so I can work and I have nurses at night so I can sleep. . . . I have NO time to care for myself.*

> *I think watching someone you love so much deteriorate is really more stress than anything in the world.*

All three of these quotes express some of the common experiences of family caregivers, feeling overwhelmed, loss of all personal time, and sadness and stress. The wife of a stroke victim wrote the first one. The mother of a severely disabled child wrote the second, and a young woman who cares for her grandmother wrote the last one.

There are certainly differences in each caregiving circumstance. A caregiver helping an elderly aunt who has diabetes will of course be dealing with different issues than a caregiver whose spouse has Parkinson's disease. These are the differences of our individual day-to-day realities and they are very real indeed. The things that separate us are the names of our loved one's diagnoses and the specific parts of the body or mind that the condition attacks.

Steven has a physical disability, but his mind is clear. The struggles of our day-to-day existence involve mobility issues and the tasks that healthy hands usually perform. Getting in and out of bed, buttoning shirts, the height of toilets and making sure the batteries that power his wheelchair are fully charged, these are our concerns. But my friend Judy had to deal with a very different set of daily circumstances when she cared for her husband who had Alzheimer's disease. Helping him remember the day of the week and what was said just five minutes ago, making sure the doors had special locks so he couldn't wander away and get lost, trying to balance caring for him and being there for her three children were the issues she struggled with.

These are very real differences, as is the fact that a wife obviously has a very different relationship with her spouse than a daughter has with her father. Your spouse is your peer, your partner, your lover. Your father helped give you life and taught you how to live it. He taught you how to ride a bike and he read you a book at night. These are the specific circumstances of relationships that affect our caregiving lives. But beneath these layers of variations, at the core of caregiving, lie the woven thread of feelings that so many family caregivers share.

I may not know what it is like to have two disabled children, as my friend Nan does, but we share similar feelings. We both know the isolation that so many caregivers describe. We can relate to the frustration that comes with caregiving, and we both know the changes, large and small, that transform our relationships in disturbing ways. We both know the sadness that comes from watching someone we love struggle to do what is a simple task for most of us. We are both very aware of the vast distance between the realities of our world and what the able-bodied healthy world thinks of as normal. We also both know the love we feel that sees past the problems we face, the inner strength we never could have imagined we had, and a view of life that is filled with both compassion and a focus on the beauty and importance of human dignity. These are the common bonds of caregiving.

Isolation

The isolation that comes from having to put so much focus on what the professionals call "activities of daily living" is compounded when friends and family turn away. So many caregivers are literally isolated from others.

A lot of people don't want to be around someone who is sick. Some friends may never call or stop by again.

Josh Sparber, Anaheim, CA

I've often wondered what it is about caregiving situations that frighten our friends away, and I've decided it is that our lives are a mirror in which they see what could possibly happen to them and their loved ones; because the picture is scary, they turn away. They don't know how to react in our presence, what to talk about, how to be with us. We can't do the things we used to do. We are less mobile, less socially nimble. Perhaps a brain injury means our spouse is no longer a charming conversationalist, or our sister has spasms and cannot talk clearly. We can't do things on the spur of the moment anymore now that mom is living with us and can't be left alone.

No one wants to think about adversity. No one wants to see it staring them in the face. And yet that is what people need to do if they are going to be our friends. They will have to put their fears aside and learn how to maneuver a wheelchair and possibly learn how to communicate with us in a new way. That's why they are friends, and we will cherish them all the more for sticking by us because we know that so many others have a hard time dealing with our changed situation and will drift away.

Diffusing Awkwardness

One way to try and prevent that from happening is to learn how to make people comfortable with your new situation. If your loved one's problems are strictly physical, perhaps he would like to be the one to explain to others exactly what is going on in his body, what limitations his condition causes and why. Fear of the unknown, discomfort with not knowing the proper way to act or what to say to someone who is different is one of the reasons that others feel awkward around us.

I recall one time when Steven and I went to see our niece Alisa, an amateur actress, perform in a play in Baltimore. Steven was using a scooter at the time. We still drove a car then, a small station wagon that allowed us to easily store the scooter in the back. After the show Alisa, her husband George, and some of their friends, who had also come to see the show that night, walked us to our car. They helped dismantle the scooter and put it in the back of the wagon and then stood around not knowing what else to do or say. Often in those days Steven's legs would go into spasm when he tried to get into the car. He'd manage to get his duff down onto the passenger seat but his legs would stiffen and shoot out in front of him, so that he was sitting facing the door instead of the hood of the car with his legs stiff and straight as wooden boards.

That night, as I tried to break the spasm so he could bend his knees and pivot to the left and be in position for me to lift his legs up and into the car, he calmly explained to the young people standing around exactly what happened and why his legs went into spasm. He told them about MS and how it stripped the nerves of their protective coating and how the scar tissue that replaced it made it very difficult, and sometimes impossible, for instructions from his brain to reach the muscles in his legs. They all listened attentively as he talked to them, and as his legs slowly lost their stiffness and became more flexible, I picked them up one at a time and put them on the floor of the car as he pivoted his body. At last he fully settled into the passenger seat, all the time keeping up the explanation. There was no awkwardness and no silent staring, which so often happens when people see someone who is disabled. The kids asked questions and you could see that they lost their initial uneasiness because of Steven's openness. I was so proud of him and how he diffused an embarrassing situation and transformed it into both an educational and comfortable one for everyone. I knew from that point onward George and Alisa would never feel awkward around us no matter how disabled Steven became, and I was right.

It Is Hard, But—

It is important to try and maintain social contacts when you are a family caregiver because it is so easy for caregiving to be all consuming. There is a book about Alzheimer's caregiving called *The 36 Hour Day*. That title is a good example of just how full your life can become when you add caregiving to an already busy schedule. Layer on top of that the physical and emotional energy drain that difficult caregiving days can bring and it is clear why we often don't have the energy to go out and party. Resting at home may well seem far more restorative than making the effort to dress and dine out with friends, and yet doing normal fun things like that is what keeps us connected, both with friends and the world beyond caregiving.

The loneliness of caregiving is ironic. We need time and energy to socialize and that's exactly what is in shortest supply when you are a family caregiver. One way to combat that is to have a friend give you a call at a scheduled time every few days or once a week. That way you are in touch with someone who cares, and since you know when the call is going to come in you can try to arrange other activities around it.

But as comforting as phone calls can be, caregivers do also need to get out of the house. If you are a working caregiver, your job may not only help pay bills, but also fulfill part of your need to socialize with others. If you can find a neighbor to go power walking with you, you can combine exercise and a chat, two things that are good for you for the price of one. Perhaps just knowing that isolation is a likely and debilitating consequence of caregiving can help you be alert enough to take steps to prevent it from getting a hold on your heart and on your life. No one ever said that life is fair, but we don't have to add the pain of isolation to our woes if we can take steps to avoid it.

Feelings of Frustration

I feel agitation, frustration, and guilt that I can't always be the victorious overcoming person I long to be.

Evelyn M. Nichols, Cedaredge, OH

I get so frustrated when he awakens me several times a night because his hallucinations are real to him.

Anna Shank, Hanover, PA

Another of caregiving's threads is the frustration we all experience because it is so hard to get things done, because non-caregivers just don't understand, because healthy people park in handicapped parking spots, and because our healthcare system isn't designed to respond to the needs of people with chronic conditions. Frustrations abound at every turn.

My friend, Evie, who is a highly resourceful caregiver, says she reaches her frustration limit when equipment breaks or doesn't function the way it is supposed to. A longtime caregiver for her quadriplegic husband, Bill, Evie tells the story of the company sales rep who told her over the phone that the lifts his company manufactured to help transfer a non-mobile person from bed to wheelchair never break, while she stood there in her bedroom with a broken bolt in her hand and the lift in pieces on the floor. "My first reaction was to scream at the guy" she said, "but then I realized I would get more help if I didn't rant and rave, but rather told him in no uncertain terms how I needed him to fix my problem."

It isn't possible to get rid of all the frustrations in our lives, whether we are caregivers or not, but a way I have found to lessen my frustration is to decide what is really worth getting upset about and what isn't. A former colleague of mine named Jim had a great way of deciding what was really important. He'd ask, "Is it worth falling on your sword for?" What a powerful way to say "pick your priorities." If we are going to let every inconvenience, every snub, get under our skin, we'll constantly be frustrated. Better to decide where to put our psychic energy and what to let go of.

One of the things that frustrates me is the inconsiderateness of healthcare professionals, especially because they should know better. Time and again when Steven goes to a doctor we are left to figure out on our own how to get him up on the examining table. They see Steven in his wheelchair and know that he can't maneuver on his own, but nevertheless do nothing to help. They just walk out of the room. I then have to go and find some people to assist us, and there aren't always appropriate people around. It sure would be nice if they had their staff make arrangements to accommodate us.

Another of my hot buttons is the same as Evie's—equipment problems. Because we rely so completely on Steven's power wheelchair in order to have a life, we are both thrown into a tizzy when it isn't working right. One way to counteract this frustration is to find an absolutely fabulous home medical equipment company that will actually send a technician out to the house to try and fix the problem right there, a wheelchair doctor who makes house calls. They do exist, although unfortunately not in every community. It doesn't stop the fact that something can go wrong, but it does give us the confidence that the problem will be fixed quickly and properly, and with a minimum of hassle.

I could make a whole list of the things that frustrate me including, at times, Steven, but I purposely try to keep my list short. After all, you can't go down on your sword every time someone is inconsiderate or the pharmacy can't fill your prescription because the pills you need are out of stock. No, we can't remove frustration from our lives; if we could we'd be living in Eden, but we can try to lessen its hold on us. One way is to plan ahead; another is to think about our most serious problems and try to find some solutions that will at least make them shrink and, ideally, go away altogether.

Frustration is an exhausting emotion. It enervates us, takes away our equilibrium. The only way it can have a positive effect on our lives is if it prods us to get rid of its cause. Since there is no way we can always do that, we must try and remember to pick our battles and decide what issues are worth going down on our swords for. That might help us feel less like wounded warriors, more of the time.

Changing Family Dynamics

My role as a wife has changed to Mommy of a once humorous, bright, and articulate husband.

Susan Kiser Scarff, Phoenix, AZ

What's the hardest thing about being a family caregiver?
Changing roles from being the child to being the one in control.

Anna Shank, Hanover, PA

The upheaval of changing family dynamics that occurs because life has been turned upside down is something that all
family caregivers can relate to. The changing relationships
often catch us off guard. We spend so much time and energy
dealing with the tasks of caregiving, getting over the emotional shock, or grieving over our losses that we often don't see
how our caregiving responsibilities are taking time away from
the other people we love. The relationship does usually change
between caregiver and care receiver, but it can also change between us and our friends and siblings and a host of others, as
well. The dynamics that accompany the decline in someone's
health or a sudden change in circumstances are complex and
disturbing. It's no wonder we don't recognize them until
they've caused a rift and are getting in the way, not only of our
ability to be effective caregivers, but also of our very happi-
ness.

Not all the changing family dynamics in caregiving families
are negative ones, some surveys have found that caregivers and
care recipients build closer bonds. In some families, first there
is a ripping apart, then a new closeness. Regardless of whether
the effects are negative, positive, or a combination of both, the
fact that caregiving affects family relationships cannot be de-
nied.

My daughter moved home [to help with caregiving for her dad].
This is a big help because she is very aware of how I feel and
the need for me to talk. She has been a wonderful source of
support.

Frances Rouse, Streetsboro, OH

My mom and I started to grow closer some years ago after
she became a caregiver for my dad. He had a stroke that left

him incontinent, slightly demented, and with embarrassing exaggerated tendencies, such as a penchant for taking things from the local Office Depot. Mom and I began to speak virtually every day as compared to our traditional pattern of once a week. She'd ask my advice. She would pour out her heart, tell me about her fear and her embarrassment over my dad's actions. I would try to comfort her and make what I hoped were helpful suggestions. I arranged home care for Steven so I could go to Florida and be with her and my dad more often. We conversed on a level we never had before, very much peer to peer, each having a better understanding of the other's personality, the other's pain, than we ever could have if we both weren't caregivers. This past year, when I went through a particularly difficult bout of depression, she sent me a greeting card every day, sometimes twice a day, to remind me I was loved, to tell me I was special, to let me know that there would be brighter days ahead. I kept them all on the mantle, even when they were stacked three deep, until she came for a visit. I wanted her to know how much I appreciated them, how much they helped. My dad is now gone and Mom has more freedom to come and visit. I enjoy her company when she is here. We are still very definitely mother and daughter, but in some ways we are sisters too, and I kind of like that.

Some people talk about role reversal when referring to a situation in which an adult child is caring for a parent, but I think that's wrong. We aren't reversing our roles. We aren't really becoming our parents' parent. We are helping them as they age in ways they used to help us, but if they have all of their faculties we must remember they have the right to make their own decisions, whether we agree with them or not. We can guide and advise them. They can ask more of us than they ever did in the past, and we can see them in a weakened condition that is antithetical to the image we had of them when we were kids, but we can never change the fact that they are our parents and we are their children.

The changing nature of relationships in caregiving situations is a touchy one. Can you still view your husband as a lover if you have to wipe his bottom every day? Can you still love your sister if she refuses to help care for your mother, especially if you are making many sacrifices to do so yourself? Will your marriage survive the pain of having produced a child with mental retardation? Will the other kids accept and love their new sister, even though she is different? These are very difficult questions. They force us to confront the very fabric of who we are as human beings. They test our compassion and our commitment and our feelings for another. Burying them under a rug will not make them go away. We need to examine them, perhaps go into therapy individually or as a family, to help us deal with them. Unfortunately they won't just go away on their own.

Tⱨe Oŋgoiŋg Sadŋess aŋd Grief of Caregivers

Perhaps the two most difficult aspects of caregiving to deal with are the ongoing sadness and grief that haunt caregivers' lives and the different reality that exists between caregiving families and non-caregiving families.

One of the most difficult emotions of caregiving is the intense sadness we feel because we love someone whose life is challenging, who hasn't been given the same chance as others, whose vigor has been taken away, or whose mental functioning has deteriorated. One of the common bonds of caregiving is the sadness that comes from wanting the miracle of wellness.

My daughter was born with such limiting disabilities that I have had to give up every dream I ever had for her.

Esther McGee, Monroe, LA

The sadness of caregivers cuts to the core of who we are as people because it touches on true grief and it ebbs and flows through our lives, sometimes right at the surface and other times buried far below. Learning to manage our sadness and grief over our losses is something that all caregivers need to do.

In one of her syndicated columns, author Ellen Goodman talked about an unwritten schedule of grief, the fact that we Americans expect things to happen quickly, that we have no patience for problems that linger, for wounds that do not heal. She said:

> The American way of dealing with it [grief], however, has turned grieving into a set process with rules, stages and of course deadlines. We have, in essence, tried to make a science of grief, to tuck messy emotions under neat clinical labels—like "survivor guilt" or "detachment" . . . We expect, maybe insist upon, an end to grief. Trauma, pain, detachment, acceptance in a year. Time's up. But in real lives, grief is a train that doesn't run on anyone else's schedule.

What do we do with this caregiver grief that never fully goes away, that doesn't have a terminus, and that may from time to time spring afresh, with new tears and new fears? I think we need to acknowledge it, for one thing. There's no reason to deny its existence. Call it by its name. Our feelings are our feelings. They are an essential part of us. Burying them only makes them change from seeds that our tears can nourish, nurture, and make grow so we can see them for what they are, into a festering mold that stays tucked away inside and eats at our inner core.

Denying our grief denies our humanity. If we didn't care, we wouldn't feel so bad. So I suggest that you take out the tissues and share your sorrow with a friend, and with your loved one, if you can. Be good to yourself. Find emotional nourishment;

get lots of hugs. Grieving is hard work. It takes time and energy. Learn from the experience so that you can grow from it, so that the grief doesn't debilitate you.

It's been over twenty-five years since Steven was first diagnosed with MS. I have dreamed new dreams. I have laughed. We have experienced the goodness of life. But sometimes the old wound aches in a certain way and I know, as I believe all caregivers know, that I am in for a spell.

When your wound hurts, whether it is still fresh or seemingly healed beneath scar tissue as mine is, remember Ellen Goodman's words—"Hearts heal faster from surgery than from loss"—and know that it is okay to cry, for yourself as well as for your loved one.

Sadness and the need to grieve are two of the threads that tie all family caregivers together. To help express these feelings and come to terms with them, some family caregivers write poetry. Sometimes they send their poetry to NFCA, and I am given the privilege of seeing inside another human being's heart.

Rita Cassidy Wiggins cares for her husband who has Alzheimer's disease. In her poem *Discovery*, she expresses the gradual grief of caregiving, the inner pain and the sadness that accompanies the progression of his disease.

> How subtly it intrudes,
> this gradual grief
> seldom visible to others,
> careful not to summon tears.
> Sometimes it seems to slip away,
> leaving just a shadow,
> barely there.
> Until one ordinary day,
> you look up and sadness is everywhere.

Jean Saucer, who cares for her mentally ill son, writes about the pain of lost dreams and the randomness with which illness strikes.

I had dreams too
confiscated by storms
and human love.
Reduced to silence
by no one's greed,
but by the winds of chance.
I dance in the spring rain
a lighting rod for thunder's pain.

Not happy poems these, but poems that reflect true feelings family caregivers experience, feelings aroused by circumstances that are outside most people's realities.

A Different Reality

Peter Dickinson is one of my favorite authors. He writes mysteries, but they are always more than mysteries. They are beautifully crafted stories that shed light on the human experience, stories that make you stop and reread a sentence two or three more times before you are willing to leave it there on the page and move on.

In his book, *Some Deaths Before Dying*, there is a sentence I've never been able to forget, perhaps because it was said by the lead character, a woman who was dying from a degenerative muscle disease and at the time of the story was bedridden, able to just move her eyelids and speak only haltingly. She had been a vibrant woman who in her healthier years had to some extent been a caregiver for her husband, a man who had been a prisoner of war during World War II and had come home bearing psychological scars. In referring to what had happened to her husband, and therefore to herself, she thought "she too had been betrayed by happenings beyond her sphere, and now she was expected to live and behave like a normal citizen, despite that."

The sentence took my breath away—"betrayed by happenings beyond her sphere, and now she was expected to live and behave like a normal citizen, despite that." Indeed isn't that what has happened to all of us who now answer to the title of family caregiver. Isn't that what has happened to the spouses, parents, partners, friends, children, siblings for whom we care? We've "been betrayed by happenings" we couldn't control and presented with the daunting challenge of trying to recreate normalcy.

It isn't an easy thing to do, recreate normalcy, when we've been hit by what feels like the equivalent of an atomic blast, and yet that is what is expected of us, and indeed what we always strive to do. But I have come to realize that, for my family and other caregiving families, normalcy is very different than it is for families that don't have to deal with disability, with the almost perverse attention to the basic acts of life that come with it and the myriad arrangements we must make to do ordinary things.

I recall once seeing a young man walking down the street. He was a wearing the typical costume of his generation, jeans and a T-shirt. Blazoned across the front of his chest in bold black letters was the statement "Normal Is Boring." I read it as he passed by me with the jaunty look of one who believes he is immortal, and I thought to myself, "He doesn't have a clue. He doesn't realize that normal isn't boring at all. It is the most wonderful thing in the world." Normal is what those of us who are family caregivers want more than anything else. We want to be like other families, to take walking and talking and eating and toileting and swallowing and thinking for granted. We want our loved one to be well. No, normal isn't boring at all, except perhaps to those who have never experienced the outside-the-norm situations of caregiving.

Steven and I have a definition of normalcy that fits our current circumstances, a definition that inevitably changes over time, as his MS continues to take its toll and impact our collective lives. These days our definition of normal includes the fact that Steven still has some strength in his legs and arms and therefore can be an active participant in helping me help him with transfers, showering, dressing, toileting, and eating. When the time comes when he can no longer do that, we will need to find other ways to deal with these basic life activities. Most likely we will need to get a lift of some sort and possibly some home care assistance. Regardless of what decisions we make at that time, the new situation will by definition become our norm, at least after the transition period from the old way of doing things to the new way is completed. What normal means for Steven and me is most likely quite different from your definition, especially if your caregiving situation is not the same as ours. How we each define normalcy isn't important, but what is important is finding a way to live comfortably with the norms that are now part of our lives, and recognize that in the world of a caregiver what's normal today may no longer be what we consider normal a year from now.

I haven't decided whether it is easier to redefine normalcy when the changes come gradually or when they come because of a more dramatic occurrence. Certainly gradual change is easier to assimilate into our lives, but it lacks the clarity of catastrophe, and doesn't always give us the opportunity to recognize the change for what it is because it sort of oozes its way slowly into our lives. But regardless of whether the changes come swiftly or slowly, they play havoc with our emotions, and we are forced to deal with what I have come to think of as the bridge between anger and acceptance.

Anger and Acceptance

Anger is an emotion we have been taught to try to hide, but these days I think of it as a very healthy emotion, one that reminds us that we are very much alive and that we burn with the fire of desire for the good things of life. Expressing our anger at the difficulties we face, the indignities we must endure, and the complex arrangements we have to make to do what should be simple rote tasks, is healthy. To rail at the gods is okay—for a time. But anger that is continuous, that can't be soothed, that lies buried beneath a calm exterior and festers like a dirty wound—that isn't healthy. Anger must eventually give way, move beyond itself to acceptance of our situation, not placid acceptance that saps our energy, but a dynamic acceptance that translates into actions that help us make the most of our transformed lives.

How do we do that? I don't think there is one set way. We must each find our own answers to that question. I can tell you about my own experience and hope there will be something in it that you can grab onto to help you move beyond any anger you may be harboring. For me it is about conscious decision-making, about making choices. The next chapter— Making Choices, Taking Charge—explores this concept in some detail, but let me say here that for me, crossing the bridge from anger to acceptance is about consciously saying, and believing, that this is where I want to be. It is about choosing to take on the responsibility of caregiving. To me that is very different from believing that I am forced to do so. I believe that despite the difficulties we confront, life awaits us. For sure it challenges us, more than it does the families of the able-bodied and mentally fit. We all wish it would challenge us less, but it is what it is, and the artistry of our lives is defined by the picture we create with our "other than normal" assortment of crayons. I am not saying it is easy. The path I walk is crooked, the bridges I cross are wobbly, and I have no idea what lies around the next bend, but I am no longer feeling that I was forced to be on this path, and that's the difference. Like the Robert Frost poem in which two paths diverge in a wood, I am choosing to walk the one less traveled. I am choosing to be a family caregiver.

My life has been "betrayed by happenings beyond my sphere" and for many years I could not accept that. But I slowly crossed the bridge and consciously chose to accept my new reality, and now with open eyes I act very purposefully and strive to "live and behave like a normal citizen." I invite you to do the same, to recognize the emotions that caregiving has evoked in you, to embrace the inner strength that comes from dealing successfully with difficult situations, and to try to move beyond the frustration, the sadness, the isolation, and the other difficult emotions that so often come with being a family caregiver. Try to look inside yourself to see if you are harboring anger, as I was. If you can recognize it, you just might be able to use that energy in a more positive way to be proactive and to take charge of your life.

A Life of Hope and Meaning

Although most of what we hear is about the dark side of caregiving, it has untold rewards as well that are best expressed in caregivers' own words.

What makes caregiving rewarding for me is the smile on his face when I walk into his room. . . . As exhausting as it is for me to be his nurse, his social worker, his advocate and his mom, all it takes to re-energize me is a few minutes at his side. Tyler's gentle caring of ME helps make it all worthwhile. He lays his hand upon my head and strokes my hair. It is calming and I think he likes being able to be the giver of care instead of the receiver.

Connie Robbins-Brady, Grand Junction, CO

As my caregiving responsibilities increased, I came to understand and accept many lessons as blessings in disguise. . . . Most of all I came to realize that caring for Sam is life itself—

that nothing I can read or study—nothing I can talk about— nothing is as important or real as simply being present with him right here, right now.

Phyllis Major, Palm Desert, CA

Caregiving is a mixed bag when it comes to our emotions. So many of the emotions associated with caregiving are dark, as we have seen, but the wonderful thing about human beings is that most of us find a hidden well of capability, strength, and resolve we never knew we had, and more often than not, we have the resiliency that teaches us how to smile through our tears.

In the end, no matter how tired, scared or worried I feel at times, I would not trade these past few years with my mother for anything. She has taught me the incredible gift of patience, acceptance, faith, and love.

Liz McLeod, Kensington, MD

Things to Think About

What feelings and emotions do you associate with your caregiving experience—frustration, sadness, grief, love, kindness, compassion, anger, pride, guilt? Have you talked to other people about them, your loved one, a therapist, another family member or friend, another caregiver perhaps? Talking about your feelings with others can really help you understand them better.

Have you considered putting your thoughts down on paper, either in a poem or in a journal? Writing poetry and journalizing are both good ways to get in touch with the emotions that caregiving arouses. They help us get underneath the crust we sometimes form as a protective coating against these emotions. Personal poems and journals don't have to be shared with anyone else. They can be your own private record of your inner self. They aren't about winning the Pulitzer Prize. They are about coming to terms with the life that the "winds of chance" have blown your way.

Recognize that you are not alone. There are millions of other family caregivers in the country who have the same thoughts and feelings that you do. There is no reason to be ashamed or embarrassed about any of your feelings. Remember that the emotions you feel are the common thread that ties you to others who care for a loved one who is chronically ill, disabled, or aged.

CHAPTER 3

Making Choices, Taking Charge

YOU are the only person who can take charge of YOUR life

Jane Hedrick, Jenks, OK

Often people become caregivers suddenly, without warning. Your husband is diagnosed with cancer and requires extensive chemotherapy. Your teenage son has a car accident and is now brain injured, unable to think clearly and respond appropriately. Your mother has a stroke that leaves her without use of her right side.

At other times, caregiving creeps up on you. You know dad is forgetting things, and you slowly start taking on some administrative tasks and calling more often, until one day you realize he no longer has the capacity to live safely on his own.

Regardless of how you became a caregiver, whether it was a terrible shock or somehow slipped up on you, in the "hubbub" of the day to day, amidst the reorientation of your schedule, the search for resources, and the fears about the future, you probably never stopped to think about exactly what happened.

You probably didn't devise a plan to help you deal with the present situation or look ahead to what the future probably had in store. If you are like most family caregivers, you just went on automatic pilot and started to do, and do, and do.

Somewhere along the line, however, it is vitally important that you stop, take a breath, and try to gain some control over the situation, rather than let the situation control you. It is vitally important that you choose to take charge of your life.

If you don't [take charge of your life], you will become bitter and resentful, and your self-esteem will ultimately suffer. You will lose sight of the reason you chose to become a caregiver in the first place, which is because you love that person and want what's best for them.

Kim Barrett, Port Orange, FL

What does that mean—choose to take charge of your life? Obviously you cannot control everything that happens to you or to your loved ones. If you could you would make their illness or disability go away. You would banish caregiving from your life and bask in the heady air of health, wellness, and "normalcy." But even though you don't have that power, you do have the power to make active choices about how you are going to deal with the caregiving circumstances of your life.

Attitude

Everything negative has a positive side. Keep on looking until you find it.

Betty S. Katz, Deerfield Beach, FL

A caregiver cannot take charge. The loved one's condition changes. . . . You can merely co-exist, maintain some sense of self, and plan for better days.

Martha Harnit, Eustis, FL

Perhaps the most important choice you have to make is how you are going to approach life from here on out. You can choose to drink the sour and acidic juice of lemons, or you can try to make lemonade out of them. You can view life as a glass that is half empty or one that is half full, and if you choose the latter view you will inevitably be a happier and healthier person. You will also be a more peaceful and loving caregiver, and more capable of proactive action on behalf of yourself and the person you care about and for.

That's because attitude impacts action. Our inner thoughts propel our outward movement. If you put on the mask of self-pity then you'll shoot a hole in every idea or suggestion that well-meaning people offer. If you wallow in the waters of negativity, you just may drown. I know. I wallowed for a very long time and I paid the price in multiple ways.

Just fake it! Act as if . . . then it makes it easier to be cheerful. Soon, you will actually feel positive. It's a decision, not a feeling.

Nancy James, Odessa, TX

I'm not suggesting that you be a Pollyanna. That doesn't make any sense either. Complete denial of your changed situation has as many negative side effects as wearing a hair shirt. What I am suggesting is that you recognize that you do have choices. They may be more difficult choices now that you are a family caregiver and have a loved one dependent on you in ways you never imagined. It is also true that some of life's options you always thought you had may now be closed to you and your family, but life still offers options and choices, and recognizing that will help you have a life that is rich and good and full, albeit in different ways than it was before. So much depends on your attitude.

Evie, the friend I mentioned before, is the perfect example of a family caregiver who revels in life and always finds its silver lining. She refers to herself as a realistic optimist. She says:

> *I have always believed that all the information we need and want is out there in the universe. But it doesn't just appear. You have to believe it is there and make the effort to find it. You have to believe that flowers can grow from rocky soil.*

I must admit I'm not like Evie. At times I tend to see the negative side of situations first. I can't immediately see the good that comes out of the bad, the rainbow after the downpour. That's why it is so good to have a friend like Evie. She can always help me see things through a brighter lens.

A positive attitude requires constant attention and practice

Judy Black, Portland, OR

How do you view your glass, as half empty or half full? Caregiving may bring forth a common grab bag of emotions, but how we deal with them is very much up to the individual and reflects our attitude toward life in general.

A year after Cindy and I went on our respite to the beach we were fortunate enough to have the opportunity to go again, but at the last minute she had to cancel, so I went by myself, which wasn't an easy decision to make, but I'm glad I did. I needed to do some thinking, some soul searching, and this gave me the opportunity.

It was a rather sad time for Steven and me because he had recently gotten his first wheelchair, the scooter no longer being sufficient for his needs. Although the wheelchair definitely made our day-to-day life easier, it was a symbol of his growing disability. It caused the old emotional wound that started with the diagnosis to reopen, and so once again I had to confront my fears about disability and our future, my sadness and my pain, and Steven had to confront his as well.

While at the beach sitting on the sand and soaking up the

warm rays of the sun, alone with my thoughts and feelings, I wrote a poem that was inspired by of all things, a beach chair. The poem erupted out of my brain in only a few minutes, and poured onto the writing pad that was propped up against my thighs. It was a very dark poem, reflecting all the painful emotions the purchase of the wheelchair engendered. It expressed my fears and my anger. It was the visible representation of the pain that I held inside. It was a poem written by a woman who definitely saw her glass as half empty. The sun was shining. I was enjoying a respite, and I decided to try and think about Steven's need for the wheelchair in a different way. I ripped up the first poem and began again. The poem that came from my inner core the second time around was more upbeat. It looked at the doors that the wheelchair opened for Steven and me, not the ones that it had closed. This is the poem I called *The Chair*, but wonder now if I should rename it *Life Depends on Your Point of View*.

It sits there at the crest of the beach, on the rise just before the sand dips towards the water's edge. A lone beach chair, seemingly abandoned.

It's a jaunty chair with its yellow striped canvas seat and sailboats floating on its blue and yellow back support. It lists just a bit to the left, almost rakishly, as it nestles in the sand, surveying the sea.

It is a chair made just for sitting, and sitting on the sand at that. It has no legs to get in the way of stretching out, relaxing, and letting the sun seep into your bones and warm your soul.

It is so unlike another chair I know. A black chair with wheels. A chair that does not survey the vastness of the ocean with a jaunty air, but rather a chair that defines a narrower kingdom.

And yet, I think this other chair is a happier chair than the one that sits and stares out to sea, for it is a chair with wheels that take the place of legs no longer able to propel their owner forth.

This other chair is not made for sitting and looking at the world. It is a chair built for exploring, for meeting life face to face and tasting of its spirit.

Perhaps this chair should have a seat of yellow and white stripes, and a back support adorned with sailboats.

A far better statement of its adventurous and joyous possibilities.

Nothing had changed in the hour between the time I wrote the first poem and the time I wrote the second one, nothing except my attitude. And yet that was everything.

Take Charge Activities and Coping Strategies

It's a fallacy of course to believe that we are ever in complete control of our lives. So much happens because of situations well beyond our ability to affect them; yet they affect us, sometimes for the good and sometimes for the bad. A big rise in the stock market can mean you'll have enough money to send your kids to college. A tornado can destroy your home beyond repair. We have no control of these circumstances, but there are others over which we do have control. We can choose where to go on a vacation, or choose to put ourselves on a low salt diet to control high blood pressure. A loved one's illness or disability generally falls into the first category, and we struggle to find ways to control its impact on their life, on our own, and on the lives of the rest of the family. We need to find ways to regain some of the sense of control that we've lost. We need to learn how to cope.

A Personal SWOT Analysis

Have you ever heard of a SWOT analysis? It is something that is done in the work world to assess a company or organization's ability to change or move forward. It is often one of the first steps in strategic planning. SWOT stands for strengths, weaknesses, opportunities, and threats. To get a handle on your life as a family caregiver, to begin to take charge, to find ways to cope with your fears, to determine what choices you have, consider conducting your own personal SWOT analysis.

We all have strengths and weaknesses. These characteristics are intrinsic to who we are. Some of them may be physical, some intellectual, some an innate part of our personality. They may change over time, or a perceived strength may be an asset in one situation and a liability in another.

Have you ever thought about your strengths and weakness in terms of your caregiving situation? If you haven't done it yet, consider making two lists. List number one can enumerate what you see as your strengths and what impact each one has, or could have, on your ability to be a successful family caregiver. List number two includes your perceived weaknesses and the consequences they have, or could have, on your caregiving. These lists can help you sort out in which areas you could really use some assistance or advice.

In my case I'd say some of my strengths are that I tend to be proactive and want to plan ahead. I can be persuasive. I can laugh at myself. I usually catch onto things fairly quickly. I don't have a problem asking for help. And I am physically stronger now than I have ever been in my life.

In terms of weaknesses, I am a five-foot one inch, small-boned woman, and although Steven is an average size man, I just don't have the leverage to help him if he falls or needs other significant physical assistance. I am lousy at math. My eyes glaze over when it comes to filling out forms. And I can be impatient, especially when dealing with bureaucracy.

Opportunities and threats come from the outside. A retirement community is being built two miles from your house, or your husband's employer will let him work from home two days a week. These are obviously opportunities that in the right circumstances could be the answer to your prayers. Threats can range from a potential loss of health insurance to the fact that you live in an old two-story house that would require extensive, and expensive, renovation to make it handicap-accessible.

Can you think of what opportunities you currently can take advantage of, or what threats you need to find ways to work around or somehow get rid of? A personal SWOT analysis is a place to begin to think about questions such as these, and it is one of the arrows in your quiver of resources to help you take charge of your life. Think of it as a "living document," one that will change as you and your circumstances do. It can be a useful tool throughout your caregiving career, not just at the outset.

Being Proactive Versus Being Reactive

Knowing more about yourself and the circumstances that could have an immediate effect on your situation is a start, but taking charge of your life shouldn't end there. Above and beyond gaining an understanding of what you bring to your caregiving situation, there are other actions you can take to give you a greater sense of ease. It is important to remember that although you can't control everything that happens, you do have the power to choose your responses and whether you are going to let circumstances take control of you or you are going to take control of circumstances.

You can be proactive or reactive regarding the caregiving needs of your family. For instance, are you going to try and educate yourself about your loved one's condition and your rights as a healthcare consumer so you can play a real role as a member of the healthcare team? Or, are you going to accept the information provided to you as gospel without asking questions or trying to insert yourself into the healthcare process?

Are you going to be proactive and do some planning, such as getting appropriate legal paperwork in order so that you can lessen the possibility of crises occurring that could be avoided? Are you going to try and learn some skills that will make caregiving a safer process for you and your loved one? There are a variety of ways you can choose to take charge of your life. Research, planning, and skill development are just three of them. Don't assume you have to do all of these simultaneously or all by yourself. Part of the process of taking charge is prioritizing and coming up with a game plan. Your SWOT analysis can play a role.

Research Takes Many Forms

Not knowing is being lost.

Rhonda Huffman, Toledo, OH

For many people anticipating becoming family caregivers, or those newly thrown into it, one of the first things they want to do is learn about their loved one's condition. Having a base of knowledge about the diagnosis can put you in a better position to ask the doctor meaningful questions about treatments, side effects, and prognoses, and also help you better evaluate recommendations given. Do you know some of the common terminology that is associated with your loved one's condition? What kind of research can you do that will increase your knowledge base and with it your confidence?

One place to go for information is a voluntary health agency (VHA) which is the general term for organizations like the American Heart Association, the Prevent Blindness Society, and the Brain Injury Association. VHAs focus primarily on finding a cure or treatments for the particular illness or condition they represent, but depending on their size and their mission, many provide all sorts of services to help patients cope with their diagnosis and its impact. In the past few years, some VHAs have begun to recognize that their sphere of concern needs to include family caregivers as well as patients, and consequently your research may turn up information and programs specifically designed to help you cope with, and become more capable at, the job of family caregiver. In the resource section of this book there is a list of many VHAs, their web sites, and their toll free phone numbers.

The Internet, of course, is the place of choice to do research these days. You can read articles written for the professional community, chat with others in similar circumstances, post questions for a doctor, create a medical journal for your loved one, stay up on the latest legislative activities that impact services for those with physical and mental disabilities, and have a conference with other members of your family. The list of what you can find out and what you can do on the Internet is seemingly endless. Information is empowering, and, generally speaking, the more you have the better off you are. I'm not an Internet whiz kid. If the truth be known, I find it rather daunting. Nevertheless, when I want and need to know something about MS, I get on-line and search away. I now know the address of some specific MS sites, but at the beginning I just went to a search engine and typed in MS. A list of sites to look at popped up. If you are just getting started, that's what I would suggest you do. Don't have access to the Internet? I bet someone you know does and they'd be happy to help out in this way.

The Internet has been my lifeline to the information I need.

Janet L. Kieffer, Mingo Jct., OH

Several years ago, when Steven started having difficulty urinating and a visit to the doctor suggested this was probably a long-term problem, I immediately turned to the Internet to learn more about his condition. We were very aware that incontinence is a big problem for many people with MS, but we'd never heard of anyone who suffered from urine retention. It never entered our heads that MS could cause someone to be unable to pee. After a couple of hours in front of the computer, I surely wasn't an expert on the issue, but I knew enough to talk intelligently to the urologist and to ask reasonable questions. I even happened on a research article he wasn't aware of. Talk about a sense of confidence! Let me tell you, when I faxed that article to him I felt so much more capable as an advocate and a family caregiver. And it was amazing how differently the doctor began to treat me. I wasn't just Steven's wife anymore, I was an important player in the discussion and decision-making process who was to be taken seriously.

Learning as much as you can about your loved one's condition is a critical activity that isn't only important at the beginning of your caregiving journey, it continues throughout the journey.

Research is a mixed bag. Obviously I read everything I can get my hands on . . . and sometimes I feel more in control. Other times, it just highlights what might be in the future and I don't always want to think about it.

Anita Bluestone, Teaneck, NJ

Research has been a big help in helping us to understand the tests that are being done and what to expect next. It helps us to make more informed decisions and feel that we still have some control over our lives and decisions.

Linda C. Jackson, Norman, OK

Rules of the Game

There's another kind of research that is equally important to do if you want to feel more in command of your caregiving life.

It's finding out the rules of the game. The world of healthcare is complex. It has its own systems of operation designed to help the medical personnel involved do their jobs, prevent injury, and maintain proper records. These systems are not designed to accommodate families.

For instance, it is important to understand that a doctor's legal responsibility is to the patient, not to you the family caregiver, unless of course you hold medical power of attorney. If you and your loved one want you to be part of the decision-making process, want you to be present during examinations and tests, then it is your loved one, assuming he or she is mentally and physically able, who must communicate that to the doctor.

Just as the medical profession has its rules, so do physicians' offices. And as with any other business, rules differ from one office to another. A good way to find out how a doctor's office works is to get to know the office staff. Learn people's names. It goes a long way toward creating a relationship as opposed to just an exchange of information. The office manager or nurse can tell you the best time of day to reach the doctor by phone, what days and hours the office tends to be busiest, what procedures must be followed if you need a prescription refill, and even the lead time involved if you want to make an appointment for a routine exam. If you know how the office is run, you are in a much better position not to find yourself in frustrating situations.

The same is true in emergency rooms and when someone is admitted to the hospital. There are procedures, and in some cases actual rules, that must be followed there. For instance, in the ER, especially if it really is a dire emergency, your job is to provide necessary information quickly and then get out of the way. In the hospital, I have found that providing a typed list of Steven's critical information is immensely helpful for the medical personnel I have to interact with. It's helpful for me too. I try to update it periodically and always take a copy of it and Steven's Living Will and Power of Healthcare Attorney with us on any hospital visit. Forms for compiling medical information exist on the Internet. I just typed up my own sheet, although at some point I plan to transfer it to a ready-made form. The list that Steven and I use includes the following:

Medical Information Form

Name and Address: Steven Mintz

Home Phone:

SS#:

Insurance:

Medical Issues: Mr. Mintz has multiple sclerosis.
                       He requires urinary catheterization.
                       He has no other medical conditions, but there is a history of diabetes in his family.
                       He has no known allergies or adverse reactions to medications.
                       His father is deceased (heart failure).
                       His mother is still alive.

Blood Type: O Positive

Care Issues: Mr. Mintz is in a wheelchair. He requires help with all activities of daily living.
                       He cannot transfer on his own. To get him onto a hospital bed or gurney, two people are needed, one to pick him up under his arms and the other to lift him beneath the knees.

Mr. Mintz's fine motor skills are greatly impaired. It is best to assume that he cannot manipulate anything on his own, except perhaps the emergency buzzer.

There is not someone at home 24 hours a day to help Mr. Mintz. After a hospital stay home care help is needed to assist with all ADLs.

Doctors:

Names/Phone Numbers:

Primary:

Specialists:

Ongoing Medications:

Names and Dosage:

Call in an Emergency:

Documents: Mr. Mintz has a Living Will.
Mr. Mintz has a Medical Power of Attorney designating Mrs. Mintz as his surrogate when necessary.

Note the detail under Care Issues. You'd be surprised how little doctors, and even nurses understand about the limits of people with disabilities, which are, of course, compounded when they are ill.

Being prepared to work within the system, or being aware of what you will face if you try to buck it, is important information to have so that you are on a level playing field with the professionals with whom you need to interact. There's nothing more unnerving or confidence deflating than to believe you are the only actor in a drama that hasn't seen the script, and if you think about it that is exactly the situation you face in healthcare settings. Everyone you will meet has been trained and in many cases licensed or certified to do their job. They are familiar with the procedures and rules. You and your care recipient are the only ones working in the dark. That being the case, the more questions you can ask, the more organized you can be, and the more you act like a healthcare advocate, the more confidence and control you will have over your caregiving circumstance.

Peer Knowledge

By doing research, I also have found other people willing to share their specific experiences, and I know that I am not alone. I have found that I am also able to help other people by sharing the knowledge that I have acquired.

Judy Horner, Boardman, OH

Some of the best research you can do involves talking to other caregivers. Learning from those who are somewhat further along on their journey than you and your loved one, or have actually completed it, can save you countless hours of effort and provide you with very concrete and practical advice.

There are many products and services available to help caregiving families, but most of us don't know what they are or where to find them, and there's no one place to go that has all the answers. Developing friendships with other family caregivers or caregiving families can enhance your ability to find what you need.

My friend Joan isn't a family caregiver. She is a person with a disability and she lives on her own. Joan has a very bad case of rheumatoid arthritis. She has had to revamp her entire life because of her illness and therefore she has searched for and found many products to help make her life easier. Although her illness is very different than Steven's, they have some of the same problems. Joan has a hard time picking up a glass because her fingers are so curled and inflexible. Steven has a hard time picking up a glass because his hands are weak and he has little sensation in his fingers. Joan told us about these extra long straws that she uses. They can be easily cut to whatever length necessary to meet your particular needs. She gave Steven one to try and told us how to get them if we were interested. We find them so helpful that we even keep some in the backpack that we take with us whenever we go out. These straws provide a very simple solution to what is actually a rather big problem, but we never would have known they existed if it wasn't for Joan. Sure, we may have come upon them if we went on a search for a product to help Steven drink from a glass more easily, but we hadn't yet begun to do that, and how much nicer to have a product be recommended by a friend who already knows that it works—and how much easier for us.

If the shoe were on the other foot, if we knew about the straws and thought they might be beneficial to Joan, we would have told her about them. When we find a superior product or service, Steven and I jump at the chance to share our finding with others. It's part of the unspoken bond that those of us outside the norm make to help each other maintain as much normalcy and independence as possible. So don't hesitate for a second to ask other caregivers or someone you might know who has a disability if they know a physical therapist they swear by, or if they know of a product that makes it easier for a person with limited mobility to get in and out of a car. It might just save you a lot of time, and effort, and anguish.

Doing research, all kinds of research, is definitely one of the ways you can begin to gain some control over your caregiving situation and improve your own sense of confidence and competency in the bargain. If research isn't your forte, if it seems beyond you regardless of the medium being used, perhaps there is someone else in your family, a friend or colleague, or a member of your congregation who can do it for you. Don't think you have to do everything yourself. Learning to be a manager, to delegate tasks, can help you feel more in control. Thinking of alternatives when roadblocks are put up in front of you is yet another way to begin to take charge of your life. It is a proactive approach to problem solving.

Planning

If you have a plan, you can enjoy what you have at the moment without as many distracting fears about the future.

Victoria Kellerman, Parkville, MD

Since becoming a family caregiver, have you done any financial or legal planning, or even sought advice about these issues? Have you evaluated your finances to see if there is any way you can afford to pay for some help? Have you tried to find out if your family is eligible for free or low cost services through local, state, or national programs? Does your loved one have a will and a living will? Do you? Do you know what Medicare does and does not cover or, if your care recipient is under sixty-five, what your private insurance will pay for? Are you aware of what might happen as your sister's condition deteriorates, and have you at least thought about what that might mean in terms of her ability to continue living on her own? Have you considered the possibility that you could have an accident or get sick? It is amazing how many questions arise when you begin to think about "what if."

I am positioning myself professionally to be able to work from home and earn the same, if not more income, if it should become necessary.

T. Mikki Crawford, Silver Spring, MD

*If anything should happen to me, what happens to my hus-
band?*

Sonia J.F. East, Copper Hill, VA

I had dinner the other evening with a colleague from out of
town who will be moving to the D.C. area shortly. Chuck con-
fided to me that his wife has a degenerative brain disorder that
was currently affecting her mobility and fine motor skills, so
it was important to him to find a house that was either all on
one level, or at a minimum had the master bedroom and bathroom on the entry floor. He wasn't sure if his wife would ever
lose her ability to climb stairs, but he thought it foolhardy to
look for a home that wouldn't easily accommodate his wife's
long-term needs. Chuck was being realistic about the future
that he and his wife could possibly face, and so he was taking
that potential future into account when making a long-term
housing investment. He was not planning that she would
definitely be unable to walk, he was planning for "what if."

As Chuck told me this, it brought back memories of when
Steven and I went looking for our current home. It was in 1987
and although Steven definitely had mobility problems he was
still able to negotiate stairs. Despite that we did exactly what
Chuck and his wife did. We thought it a realistic possibility
that Steven wouldn't be able to climb stairs at some point in
the future and so we only looked at one-story homes. In fact
we went on our search with a very specific accessibility checklist in hand. It included a shower stall in the master bedroom,
easy access to the backyard and a garage that had, or could
have, an automatic garage door opener. The house we bought
didn't meet all the criteria on our checklist but it met most of
them. Over the years we've made some changes to accommodate Steven's growing disability, and although some of them
required a bit of ingenuity, they were all doable because we
planned ahead.

None of us can plan for all of life's possibilities, but we can definitely plan for some of them. I know from experience how emotionally difficult it is to look ahead toward what your caregiving might entail in the future. Nevertheless, it is very prudent to do some forecasting because if you don't, your life may well be filled with many more crises than it needs to be. Being part of a caregiving family is hard enough as it is. There's no point in making it harder than it has to be. Planning for the future can help put you in the driver's seat of life and also help ward off situations that make you feel dependent.

At each step we have tried to anticipate the next problem dad would be facing. . . . In talking with dad's doctor about what to expect, we were plugged into hospice early. . . . This forward thinking has helped us not have to scramble and has helped us be mentally prepared as changes occurred.

Lois Finnan, Newburgh, IN

It's been said that Americans are the only people on the face of the earth who think death is negotiable. I don't know if that's true, but I do know that we have a very hard time talking about death and therefore planning for it. That's the one thing we can, and should, all do, even if caregiving isn't part of our lives.

Some years ago I had the wonderful opportunity to play a leading role in an extraordinary public education campaign to change the way we as Americans think about, and deal with, end of life issues. The program, Last Acts, which is still ongoing, is a multimillion-dollar effort funded by the Robert Wood Johnson Foundation, one of our nation's leading philanthropic organizations focused on healthcare issues.

Last Acts has created a quiet revolution that is changing the practice of medicine in terms of how it treats pain. It is raising the public's awareness of end of life issues by working with Hollywood producers to include end of life scenarios in major TV shows, such as ER. And it is teaching us that death is a natural part of life that we can and should plan for, and that although death is not pleasant, a family can experience it in a calm and loving way.

You may think this is morbid, but in fact it is one of the most life-affirming things you can do. What a great gift to allow someone you love to complete their life on their own terms!

Caregiving Skills

I have learned to insert/remove the catheter to remove blood clots and relieve my father's pain quickly. I no longer have to call the doctor or take him to the hospital for this.

Jane Hedrick, Jenks, OH

In addition to research and planning there are other things you can do to feel more secure in your actions and therefore more in charge of your life. You can learn some specific skills that help you be a more capable and confident family caregiver. For instance you can learn how to communicate more effectively with healthcare professionals, above and beyond knowing the terminology associated with your loved one's diagnosis. You may want to learn nursing techniques and skills that make tasks easier for you and your loved one, or some of the basic skills that physical therapists, special needs teachers, and other professionals go to school to learn and get licensed to do. When we realize all the things there are to learn to be comfortable and confident in our caregiving role, it's no wonder we so often feel out of our depth. Half of the caregivers in a recent NFCA survey of family caregivers said they hadn't been properly trained to do the caregiving work they were currently doing, so you certainly aren't alone if you are feeling unprepared.

I have become proficient with the laws and rights of the disabled community and make it a point to inform others.

Cynthia J. Cavallaro, Swampscott, MA

There isn't one magic place to go to learn skills that can help you in your caregiving. Some hospitals do provide training programs, so it is worth checking with the ones in your community. If your loved one is eligible for home care services, the agency providing them can certainly teach you skills and techniques as well. Make sure you know what your insurance will and will not cover. Some policies allow a set number of visits by an occupational therapist or physical therapist if ordered by a doctor, and these professionals can teach you transfer techniques and other life skills. Don't forget the voluntary health agency focused on your loved one's condition or the Red Cross chapter in your community.

I went to my local college and became a licensed nursing assistant.

Janet L. Kieffer, Mingo Jct. OH

Managing Instead of Doing

Research has shown that men approach caregiving differently than women. Whereas women tend to jump in headfirst and do everything themselves, men tend to take more of a managerial approach and delegate or purchase outside services. Regardless of whether you are a man or a woman, you can learn how to manage your caregiving responsibilities as opposed to letting them manage you. A professional geriatric care manager may be able to help you do just that and actually assist you in finding the right solution to meet your loved one's needs and your own, as well. Whether your loved one is elderly or not, consider learning some care management skills. Here are some tips from the professionals.

1. Educate yourself on the nature of the disease or disability you're dealing with. Understanding what is happening to your care recipient will make you better able to judge the kind of resources you'll need.

2. Write down your observations and evaluations of your care recipient's personal strengths and weaknesses, as well as the physical and/or mental deficits caused by their condition. This assessment will not only help you come to a realistic view of the situation, it will be a handy baseline reference to chart the progression of symptoms and changes. It's also not a bad idea to write down your own strengths and weaknesses so you can be realistic about your own need for help and support. If you have impairments of your own, i.e., a weak back or high blood pressue, list those as well.

3. Hold a family conference and decide who will handle which chores if more than one family member is involved. Making sure everyone knows his or her responsibilities keeps misunderstandings to a minimum and saves one person from bearing the brunt of all the work. Be aware that family meetings work best when there is a third party there to facilitate them. It could be a care manager, a member of the clergy, a long-standing family counselor, or anyone who can be trusted not to "take sides" and also has the skills to keep the meeting on topic, on schedule, and all parties feeling safe so they can truly say what is on their minds.

4. Keep good records of emergency numbers, daily medications, special diets, back-up people, and other pertinent information relating to the care of your loved one. Update as necessary. This record will be invaluable if something happens to you.

5. Research services in your area, including respite care, adult day care, nursing facilities, volunteer programs, and churches. Look at them from a dual viewpoint— which ones are there to help your care recipient, which ones exist to help you or both you and your loved one.

6. Join a support group or find another caregiver with

whom to converse or correspond. In addition to emotional support, you'll be likely to pick up practical tips.

7. Start advance planning for difficult decisions that may lie ahead. It's much tougher to think decisions through when and if the situation turns desperate. Don't neglect to discuss wills, advance directives, and powers of attorney. These instruments give care recipients the opportunity to make their wishes known, but they can be signed only when a care recipient is competent, so it's best not to delay.

8. Develop your own support system. Be willing to tell others what you need and to accept their help.

9. Establish a family regimen. When things are difficult to begin with, keeping a straightforward daily routine can be a stabilizer, especially for people who find change upsetting and confusing.

10. Approach some of your hardest caregiving duties like a professional. Instead of seeing yourself as a spouse or child, step back and try to insulate yourself from the sense of loss such duties evoke in you, concentrating instead on the practical aspects of getting the job done as efficiently as possible. Sometimes your best defense is to distance yourself a bit so you can accomplish the difficult tasks without allowing them to take a constant emotional toll.

These are just a few of the ways you can begin to take charge of your life now that you are a family caregiver. It's all about incremental steps and small things that make a difference. Remember, small steps over time can add up to big accomplishments and a significantly different sense of self-esteem and capability. These two personal strengths can help you feel more on top of things, especially if you can keep your cup of attitude at least half full.

CHAPTER 4

Caregiving Is About Love, Honor, Value—and You

Rabbi Hillel, one of the great sages of Judiasm, is the author of my favorite quote. He said:

> If I am not for myself, who will be for me?
> If I am only for myself, what am I?
> And if not now, when?

I know of course that Rabbi Hillel, who lived at the time of Jesus, wasn't thinking about those of us who are family caregivers today, but when I first read these lines, it seemed to me that his words transcended time and took on new meanings for each age, and that for our age, his message applied to family caregivers.

So often we are not for ourselves. On the contrary, we give and give and give to help another. No wonder non-caregivers often refer to us as saints or angels. We have no problem living up to the implications of Hillel's second question.

It is his first question that we have a hard time taking to heart. We tell ourselves we need to get more exercise and more sleep, and we need to find more opportunities to relax or take a respite break. Hillel's first question causes many caregivers to laugh and say, "Yeah, right. I'm going to drop everything now and meet my friends for a cup of coffee or go for a bike ride."

The rabbi's words can actually be a wake-up call for all family caregivers, if we allow ourselves to recognize that self-care isn't a luxury but rather a necessity that can actually improve our ability to provide high quality care for our loved one. They can serve as a reminder that loving yourself is not selfish, but rather is a way of honoring and valuing the wonder of human life.

The Gift of Good Health

Why is sometimes acting in your own behalf such a valuable thing to do not only for yourself, but also for your loved one? The answer is actually quite simple. If something happens to you, if you get sick, become severely depressed, can't continue to function as a caregiver at a high level, what then will happen to the person you love and care for? Is there someone ready, willing, and able to jump in at a moment's notice and fill your place? I doubt it. What if you died? It could happen. Your own good health must be preserved if you are going to go the distance as a family caregiver.

A study published in 1999 in the *Journal of the American Medical Association* reported on a study of elderly spousal caregivers. The researchers found that those caregivers who experienced significant stress were sixty-three times more likely to die within a four year period than non-caregivers, and also more likely to die than caregivers in less stressful situations.

Other studies over the years have also documented the physical and mental repercussions of family caregiving. Depression, sleeplessness, and backaches are commonplace among family caregivers who help their loved one with personal care activities. One study, published in the English medical journal, *The Lancet,* described how family caregivers can have slower healing times than non-caregivers, the stress having a direct effect on the body's own ability to repair itself.

These are extraordinary statements. They are scary. They imply that in certain circumstances family caregivers are literally putting their lives on the line to provide quality care to someone they love. Instead of one patient, we end up with two. Just think about the dire consequences if you were bedridden for a while. Caregivers who let their own health suffer, thinking that their time is better spent caring for a loved one, are actually taking a huge risk. If you are in the hospital suffering from exhaustion, if you neglect a minor cough and it develops into pneumonia, or if you are in a serious car accident, who then will be the caregiver? Loving, honoring, and valuing yourself isn't just a nice thing to do if you have the time. It's essential.

Recently one of my daughter's physicians told me, "The worst thing that can happen to your daughter is not her health problems; the worst thing that can happen to your daughter is not having you to care for her." This confirmed and encouraged my attitude as a caregiver that my well being is my daughter's well being.

Linda Reid, Oneonta, AL

That's why every time you get on an airplane and the cabin crew recites their safety messages they always end with "if the cabin loses pressure, and you are traveling with a small child or someone else that needs assistance, put your own mask on first." Why is that such an important message? Why are we advised to help ourselves first? It is because, if we are gasping for air, how can we possibly assist someone else? Our investment in ensuring that we are breathing normally pays a large dividend to our loved ones. It gives us the capability to help them now, and it just may be the critical reason we can continue to help them in the future.

Imagine you are driving down the highway and your fuel gauge is beginning to look rather low. Eventually the warning light comes on to tell you it is definitely time to fill up with gas, and that's what you do. You stop at the next gas station rather than push on any further, rather than taking the chance of getting stuck. This is just prudent behavior that ensures our ability to keep on driving and eliminates the fear that we will run out of gas and have to call AAA.

Now compare being a caregiver to driving that car. Imagine that your energy level is near zero. You have noticed warning signs that suggest you need to refuel. You are more impatient than usual and you anger more quickly. You aren't sleeping well and your back hurts constantly. With all of these symptoms, why is it so hard for us to pull over and fill up our own tank?

There are any number of answers to that question, not the least of which is that most of us have been brought up with the American ideal of being independent. We think taking a break means we are not fulfilling our obligations to those we love, that prioritizing our need for regular exercise and a solid night's sleep implies that we are selfish. After all, a parent's job is to protect and care for his or her child. The Ten Commandments direct us to "honor thy father and mother." Wedding vows are promises made and kept. "For better or for worse" translates for some into being there twenty-four hours a day, no questions asked.

Caregiving Is About Relationships

We forget that all of these dicta imply the existence of a relationship, a relationship between at least two people and, as in all relationships, the views and needs of all parties must be taken into account if the relationship is going to be a successful one. Although family caregivers and care receivers are separate and distinct people, we are linked together in a unique way. After all, family caregivers do not exist unless someone they love needs care. And if that person should die then the family caregiver relinquishes his or her title.

This dichotomy between being an individual and being part of an inseparable relationship is often at the core of a great deal of conflict between caregivers and care receivers. I believe the conflict often stems from the fact that neither we nor our loved one recognize and come to terms with the special quality of our relationship. It is as if we family caregivers and our loved ones are Siamese twins having our own heads and our own hearts, but we are joined at the hip, and by necessity must continuously make accommodations for each other if we are going to live in harmony and get things accomplished.

If your care recipient's condition is strictly physical, then it is easy to see why and how two points of view are part and parcel of the caregiving equation. If your care recipient is developmentally delayed, mentally ill, or brain injured, there are obviously extenuating circumstances that change the balance of accommodation and decision-making, but they don't change the fact that at least two people are affected by whatever decisions are made, your care recipient and you.

Caregiving is by definition a relationship in which one person needs care and another is called on to provide it. It is about loss and challenges and finding a new balance. It's about recognizing that although one person's diminished health and ability to function independently was the catalyst for making yours a caregiving family, everyone in the family, including you, the primarily caregiver, has been deeply affected as well. A successful caregiving relationship requires that caregiver and receiver recognize that each of you has needs and rights and feelings that have to be considered, honored, and addressed in an equitable way. And although yours may be the primary relationship, it is important to recognize the impact on other close family members as well, especially children, whether they be siblings, friends, or grandchildren of the person needing care.

The way I cope best with my caregiving situation is to have enriching activities that I take part in apart from my spouse. This is extremely important for me and our relationship.

Anita Bluestone, Teaneck, NJ

I wish Steven and I had understood this back in 1974 when he was diagnosed with MS. It might have saved us a great deal of pain. We didn't understand how vitally important it was that we learn to look at the impact of his illness through each other's eyes. We do that now. In fact it has become the guiding light of our marriage and how we cope with the fact that ours is a caregiving family.

Our problem was that we couldn't communicate about MS. We couldn't get a real dialogue going about our fears, our sadness, our different ways of coping. I'm by nature a talker, a planner. Steven keeps things to himself and prefers to deal with things as they arise.

Steven is the one with the clinical diagnosis of MS, but we both are living with it. I wanted to be prepared for whatever might lay ahead. He found an internal control by trying to go along as much as possible as we always had. Our inability to recognize that we both needed very different things in order to function successfully with the MS in our lives was what led to our separations.

What got us back together and has kept us together now for more than a dozen years was the realization that we needed to find a way to satisfy both of our competing grieving and coping styles. If our relationship was to be based on equality, we had to find a way to balance our competing styles and reach a successful compromise.

I have come to understand that he needs time to deal with his own private hell, with the changes in his body, with decisions brought about not in the normal course of life, but because of the MS. I have come to recognize that Steven is a "quiet fighter" and that for him acknowledging the changes in his body means accepting that there is no turning back to a higher level of functioning. Acknowledging to himself that he needs more help is an acceptance that the MS is taking its toll. It is not an easy thing to do and he needs to do it, not in resignation, but consciously and with dignity, and in his own way.

Simultaneously, the reason he can now more easily acknowledge that there is something to be said for my point of view is because he has come to see his MS through my eyes. He's come to understand that my suggestions to look into a new piece of equipment or ask others for help is not meant to take away his independence but rather to protect his safety and to actually give us back some of the independence that his increasing disability is constantly taking away from us. He's come to understand that I too have rights when it comes to how we deal with the disability in our lives, and that indeed, for our relationship to work and to grow, we both need to give a little in order to gain a lot.

We both learned our lessons the hard way, but that is all in the past. We are stronger for the pain, and our relationship is now constructed on solid ground. This process of viewing situations through each others eyes is based on love and respect and honoring the fact that Steven's illness is our illness, that we are both affected by it but need to deal with it in different ways and along a different time continuum. It recognizes that in a relationship, a good relationship, all parties count and everyone's point of view has value.

Permission to Say "No"

Another way to love, honor, and value yourself is to recognize that even though you are a family caregiver, you don't always have to say yes to requests or demands. On the contrary, it is important to acknowledge that you don't have to discard the word "no" from your vocabulary to continue being a loving and thoughtful caregiver who provides high quality care to your loved one. "Yes, I can and will do this," and "I'm sorry, I just can't do that," are perfectly legitimate statements to make. This may sound like heresy. You may be thinking, "How can I possibly say no?" "How can I not continue to give and give when she needs me, when the doctor says these are the tasks that must be done?" The reason is that saying "no" now could in the long run provide you with the ability to say "yes I can" for a long time to come. It can help you find the balance you need between self-care and caregiving. Family caregivers don't have formal rights enacted by law, or even rights established by custom, that apply to all of us, but we all have the right, indeed the natural instinct, to self-preservation.

When doctors or other health professionals assume that you can do specific tasks or therapies or be at the hospital at a specific time to take your loved one home, they generally have no idea what your other obligations are, and unless you set them straight they will go on assuming that you can and are willing to do whatever they ask, when they ask it.

It all comes down to setting boundaries.

Lauren Agoratus, Mercerville, NJ

Ann Selby (a pseudonym), a forthright health policy analyst I know, told me how she stood up to a doctor recently when he gave her a list of instructions for caring for her dad, who had just had heart surgery, after he was released from the hospital. She said, "I told him in no uncertain terms that I had other responsibilities. I could not be at the hospital the next day to take my dad home, and I could not stay with him in his house while he was recuperating, that he [the doctor] needed to order some homecare services for my dad. He was assuming that I had no constraints on my time. He didn't consider whether I had a job or a family. When I told him he couldn't make those assumptions, and he realized I wasn't going to kowtow to him, he came up with another plan that was much more reasonable. He let my dad stay in the hospital an extra day so I could make arrangements to pick him up and wrote an order for homecare services so that an aide would come in every other day for a week to give him a bath and help with some other personal needs."

Not everyone has Ann's gumption, but at times we would all benefit if we did. A strong sense of self and a belief in what is right and wrong with our healthcare system has become a necessity for all of us who want to have some control over our caregiving situation rather than allowing the standard practices and assumptions of the medical community to add to the stress of our lives. We need at times to learn to say no.

Recognizing the need to say no is one thing; training yourself to do it is quite another. It goes against everything we have been taught about how to behave with healthcare professionals and against our natural instincts on how to help those we love, but if we are going to maintain our ability to provide care for an extended period of time, we need to know when saying no is the best thing we can do.

It involves understanding when we are "pushing the envelope," and whether we need to find a way to get some relief for our own benefit as well as for our loved one's. The lifting you could easily do five years ago, may have dire consequences for your back today. The sleepless nights you were able to rebound from in your thirties may be a serious health risk in your fifties. By honoring the rhythms of your body and your mind, you are honoring your own life and the contributions you make to your loved one's well being.

It takes a lot of courage to admit you aren't superwoman or superman and that you can't carry on the way you have in the past. When it comes to caregiving, a lot of courage and determination are needed to say no and to choose another path, even if only temporarily. Maybe that's why less than thirty percent of the respondents to a 2001 NFCA survey of self-identified family caregivers strongly agreed with the statements, "I feel comfortable saying no when asked to do more than I think I can by professionals," and "I feel comfortable saying no when asked to do more than I think I can by my loved one." Learning to say no when it comes to our loved one's requests or doctors' orders doesn't come easily. It is something we have to practice over time, and then to know when it is the appropriate response.

I know how hard it is because I've said no to Steven from time to time. The most recent time was when my doctor told me I was suffering from fatigue and anxiety. She gave me some medication to help me sleep through the night, something I hadn't done for months. I decided getting enough sleep needed to be my number one priority if I was going to be able to function successfully. And I decided that returning to a regular pattern of exercise, another "good for me" endeavor that had fallen by the wayside of caregiving, would be my number two priority.

Unfortunately, for me to do both of these things, Steven had to alter his nighttime schedule. Steven likes to stay up until at least eleven on weeknights, and even later on weekends. I like to be in bed no later than 10:30 and sometimes earlier. He is also more comfortable going to sleep on his back and then being shifted onto his side four or five hours later. I decided I couldn't do that all the time anymore. I said: "No, I need to try and get as much uninterrupted sleep as possible. I need to wake up refreshed and try to get some quality exercise at least three mornings a week. I need to take care of myself as well as of you. Because I have to help you undress and get into bed, I need you to honor my needs more than your own for a little while. In the long run we need to find an equitable compromise."

Despite the fact that Steven has MS, and each year he seems to need help with more and more activities of daily living, our relationship is still a partnership. The bonds are there, as is the closeness that comes from sharing experience, both good and bad, in an open and honest way. There is no question that I am his caregiver, but we are still husband and wife. That being the case I asked him to become my caregiver temporarily and help me restore my physical and mental balance. And you know what? He said okay, and was no worse off because of it.

The Guilt Factor

I never seem to find time for myself without wondering if she is okay.

Rosie Miller, Phoenix, AZ

The fact that I did it and he agreed doesn't mean that this was a guilt-free experience. It is one thing to understand something intellectually. It's quite another to get beyond your emotional demons. If you feel guilty when you think about caring for yourself and taking a break, you are definitely not alone. Over the years I have heard many reasons given by family caregivers as to why they couldn't take a little time just for themselves, why they couldn't spare some time to protect their own health. They include:

I'd worry all the time I was gone anyway, so why bother.
It wouldn't be right to do something just for me.
I know I should go to the doctor, but I am all doctored out.
I don't have the energy to exercise.
No one else could possibly care for John the way I do.
My mom would never let anyone else care for her.
I don't have the money to take a break.

If you feel guilty when you think about doing something that would be fun or would give you an emotional or physical boost, think about the fact that even though you are providing care because you love and feel responsible for someone, much of the caregiving that you do is in fact a job, a job that other people get paid to perform. If caregiving was your paid employment, if you were a doctor, nurse, physical therapist, short order cook, or office administrator, you would more likely than not receive at least two weeks of vacation every year, even though mandatory vacation is not required in the United States. As a family caregiver you are in essence self-employed. You aren't getting a salary and the job of caregiving doesn't provide you with health insurance, but as your own "boss" you can at least grant yourself some time off.

In Canada the law does require employers to provide employees time off, ten days of it with full pay. In the U.K. mandatory vacation is twenty-four days and in Germany, France, and Sweden it's twenty-five. That's actually good human resource policy. It makes great business sense. People are more productive when there is balance in their lives, when they take the time to "fill up their tanks." But, since this is America, and as far as your caregiving job goes you are your own boss, it's up to you to enforce a mandatory vacation rule for yourself, even if that vacation is broken up into half hour breaks every afternoon. We all need a chance to rest, a change of scenery from time to time, and we all need to enrich our lives by meeting new people. Besides, have you ever considered that your loved one might like a break from you and would appreciate seeing and talking with others?

Barry Jacobs, Ph.D., is a clinical psychologist and family therapist. He is an associate director of behavioral sciences for the Crozer-Keystone Health System in Springfield Pennsylvania, and he teaches at three universities, including the University of Pennsylvania School of Nursing and the Temple University School of Medicine. According to Dr. Jacobs, caregiver guilt has several sources, including an overpowering sense of obligation that is sometimes heightened by admonitions from other family members to keep up the good work. At times survivor guilt comes into play. What did I do to cause this tragedy? What didn't I do to prevent it? Because Mary can no longer play golf, I'll give it up too.

I can relate to all of these reasons to feel guilty. Whenever my mother-in-law tells me how wonderful I am and how much she loves me, I think about all the things I don't do that could possibly make life easier for her son. Whenever my manicurist tells me how special I am for staying with Steven, I feel as if I am being anointed with a sainthood I don't deserve. I've certainly felt guilty because I am glad that I'm not the one who has MS. And I remember a period of time when I tried to live my life at Steven's pace so as not to leave him alone or leave him out of activities. In all of these instances the guilt didn't make me feel better. In fact it made me feel worse. That's because guilt is an insidious emotion that uses up a lot of energy to no purposeful end. It just makes a difficult situation even more difficult, and it certainly gets in the way of loving, honoring, and valuing yourself.

Respite

It isn't possible to talk about self-care for family caregivers without talking about respite. More than any other service, respite is what family caregivers want most. The primary purpose of respite care is to provide relief from the extraordinary and intensive demands of ongoing care to someone with special needs, and thereby strengthen the family's ability to provide care. Respite care is planned and proactive. Respite means taking a break before extreme stress and crisis occurs.

A respite doesn't have to mean a week on the French Riviera, although that sounds pretty nice to me. It doesn't even have to be a weekend visiting friends, at least not at first. A respite can be as simple as lying on the couch with the lights dimmed listening to your favorite music, especially if you do it on a regular basis. It can be going to the movies or having a manicure every other week. You might even think of your three times a week exercise routine as a respite, if you enjoy it, rather than thinking of it as something you do because it is good for you.

I've come to think of respite as coming in three sizes, much the way things did in the house of the three bears that Goldilocks visited. The week away is obviously comparable to a "papa bear" respite. A weekend visiting friends would fit nicely into "mama bear's" bowl, and all the little things that take an hour or less can be easily categorized as "baby bear" respites.

If the truth be told, I've never taken a "papa bear" respite. The longest I've been away is four days and I had the built-in justification that it was for a business trip. But I have taken weekend respites, and each time I have reaped more benefits than I could have imagined. There was of course the weekend that Cindy and I went away and started to talk about our caregiving experiences. There was the weekend the following year when I went to the beach by myself and wrote the poem about the chair. I wrote another poem that weekend. There seems to be something about the salt air and the warmth of a summer breeze that nourishes my creative juices. The poem is called *Respite*, and I've been told that it expresses the benefits that a weekend away can bring.

> I rented a house at the beach this weekend.
> I went by myself and I took long walks.
> I sat by an inlet of the bay and watched the
> reeds and intermittent trees, while they
> danced lightly in the breeze.
> I felt the sun's warmth on my face,

and I willed it to seep deep into my soul.
I went to the beach by myself this weekend.
I was alone, but I was not lonely.
I was with my self, and we were at peace—
with each other.

It's a wonderful feeling being with your self. For me it means living in the moment, breathing slowly and deeply, feeling a delightful sense of calm and warmth.

I can achieve some of this same feeling by indulging in my favorite "baby bear" respite, a bath by candlelight. Bubbles are a delightful addition, but they are optional. There is something about the glow of the candlelight, though, that is essential to the experience because it somehow takes the edge off the responsibilities that lie just beyond the bathroom door. Warm water and soft lighting are sometimes enough for me, but at other times the addition of some calming music really helps take me away. It blocks out whatever household noises are invading my privacy and it involves yet another one of my senses in the experience. Touch, sight, sound, and sometimes taste and smell are added to my respite bath. A warm cup of tea gives me a glow on the inside just the way the warm bath water gives me a glow on the outside, and the scent of the tea, especially if it is a fruity blend, is yet another way to remove myself further from the day-to-day. And every now and then I add the pièce de résistance, a piece of good quality chocolate. It adds a sort of decadent quality to the whole experience, but that's just the point. I've come to the conclusion that if you are going to have a respite that only lasts fifteen or twenty minutes, it really should be decadent to have the proper effect.

I remember a time when I had been feeling fairly low and I mentioned it to a friend on the phone. A few days later a package arrived in the mail. When I opened it a huge smile spread across my face. Inside was a basket filled with everything I could possibly need for a delightful bathtub respite—bath oils, moisturizer, a big sponge, and lovely smelling soaps. I don't think I've ever gotten a more thoughtful gift.

You may be thinking I am mad, but the point is that it works for me. What you do on a respite break, regardless of its length, is up to you. It has to meet your needs, break your tensions, renew your spirit. It needs to be the right medicine to cure or at least ameliorate your current stress. It needs to be for you, precisely because you do so much for others, and because you deserve it.

Next time you feel guilty for even thinking about taking a break, remember it is only partially for your benefit. Your loved one will reap a great deal of the benefit, as well. Respites are guaranteed to take the edge off your tension, renew your energy, and give you a fresh dollop of patience with which to pick up your caregiving duties once again. Respite is the primary mechanism you have as a family caregiver to refill your tank and thereby keep on going. If you need proof, here it is.

Two family members volunteered to give us relief [from caring for my mom] for a week's family vacation. We had a wonderful time with our sons and came back refreshed.

Ruthann S. McDonough, Carmel, IN

A number of studies have proven the value of respite to caregivers and their loved ones. A study looking at the benefits of respite for parents of children with emotional and behavioral disorders, published in 2000, shows that respite enhanced the capacity to cope with stress, lessened the number of institutionalizations, and created greater optimism about the caregiver's ability to continue to provide care.

A study of caregivers of Alzheimer's patients published in the *Journal of the American Medical Association* in 1996 showed that respite and counseling lessen depression and help caregivers avoid nursing home placement for their loved one for as much as a year.

Practical Realities

Even if you want to take a weekend respite several times a year, or go to a weekly support group meeting, even if you truly believe self-care is a necessity and not a luxury, making it happen isn't always easy.

The survey of self-identified family caregivers revealed a disheartening fact. It found that even among family caregivers who believe strongly in the principle of caregiver self-care, there was often a disconnect between belief and action. Some of the survey questions were designed to gather data about the respondents' healthful activities both before and after becoming family caregivers. The answers to this series of questions were quite disturbing.

All of the respondents ate more nutritious meals, got more exercise, and went to see their doctor when they suspected a problem with their own health more often before becoming family caregivers than after. It wasn't because they didn't think it was important to continue these activities to the extent they had before. In fact, these caregivers said they thought it was extremely important that all caregivers be told to preserve their own health. The survey didn't explore the reasons the caregivers didn't or couldn't maintain their previous healthful behaviors, but I would surmise it was because, now that they had caregiving responsibilities, they just couldn't find the time or manage the logistics as easily as before.

My body tells me I need a break, but I can't seem to find the resources to be able to do it.

Jack Morris, Orlando, FL
(Pseudonym)

There probably isn't just one answer to these questions. I know for myself that sometimes the thought of going to yet another doctor's appointment, even if it is to make sure that nothing is seriously wrong with me, is just too overwhelming. It means more time away from work. It means being in the milieu of medicine yet again. Sometimes I'm just too bloody tired to get up and exercise. I'll shut off the alarm and hunker down under the covers for an extra thirty minutes of shut-eye, especially in the winter. It's easy to find an excuse not to do it. Life is more complicated than it used to be, time is more occupied with another's needs. Wanting to do something and then doing it are two totally different things. And the reasons you can't are at times out of your control.

Eleanor Cooney, a writer whose mother has Alzheimer's disease, angrily explains her point of view in an article in the October 2001 issue of *Harper's Magazine*:

> Stability and predictability in daily routine are what the sages prescribe for people with Alzheimer's. They also have wise words for the caregivers: Take care of yourself. Give yourself a break. Be sure to set aside time to do the things you enjoy. Get plenty of rest. Pamper yourself. Enlist the help of friends and relatives to assist with your "loved one." Take time out for yourself, they chant. Time out for yourself? I'll let you in on a secret. There is no time out, not even when you are sound asleep, if the person is in fact a loved one and money is scarce.

I suppose I am one of the sages that Eleanor is referring to. I certainly felt her anger jump off the page and punch me in the stomach the first time I read her words, and repeated readings haven't softened the blow. I understand her anger. I've had plenty of my own, but my anger wasn't focused on any particular message or human messenger as hers is. I was angry at God.

I know many caregivers, maybe some of you who are reading this book, share Eleanor's anger, and agree that I, and others who speak to and for family caregivers, are way off base. I respect your right to your anger, but I'd suggest it is misplaced.

Family caregivers do need to take care of themselves, do need time off. The problem is, as Eleanor Cooney so vividly says, that at times this seems impossible to do for both emotional and practical reasons.

Eleanor referred to the scarcity of money being an issue for her. As distressing as it is, it's not surprising. It is expensive to be a caregiving family. Surveys have shown that family caregivers tend to have lower household incomes than non-caregiving families. Thirty-five percent of the general population has an income of under $30,000. Forty-three percent of caregiving families fit into that category. Some caregivers leave the workforce. Others turn down promotions or decide to work part-time. All of this, of course, impacts income and benefits.

With most people's health insurance being part of their employment package if they are under sixty-five, the irony of being a family caregiver is that, should you leave the workforce to take on the responsibility of giving care to someone whose health is compromised, you may well be forced to compromise your ability to take care of your own. Add to that the fact that many of the products and services caregiving requires just aren't covered by either private or government insurance including items such as grab bars for the bathroom and other home modification products, non-medical transportation, and ongoing personal care. Yes, being on a tight budget can easily be one of the reasons that a family caregiver has difficulty taking time for herself or himself.

In addition to having limited finances, not having family or close friends nearby to help out can be a big factor in making it harder to "be for yourself." In some cases when money isn't the issue, finding people or services to hire is. For family caregivers something usually has to give because our society isn't geared up to help us. More often than not what gives is ourselves. My point is that you can't always let that be the case because it can have dire effects not just for you, but for the very person you are trying to care for.

We are beginning to stray into the waters of public policy

when we start to talk about income inequity and lack of services. This is neither the time nor place, but I want you to remember Eleanor's words and anger later on because I believe we need to harness that anger and use it. "Love, Honor, and Value Yourself" should never be seen as an expression created by blind idealists who don't have a clue what family caregiving is really about. Rather, it should be seen as is a simple statement of something we all believe is important and that also is, if not easy, at least doable for all of us, with some acceptable level of effort.

Permission

Robert Bly wrote a poem that knocked me off my feet the first time I read it. It is a poem of great imagination. It is a poem of permission. It is a poem family caregivers should take to heart.

Things to Think

Think in ways you've never thought before.
If the phone rings, think of it as carrying a message,
Larger than anything you've ever heard,
Vaster than a hundred lines of Yeats.

Think that someone may bring a bear to your door,
Maybe wounded and deranged; or think that a moose
Has risen out of the lake, and he's carrying on his
antlers
A child of your own whom you've never seen.

When someone knocks on the door, think that he's
about
To give you something large: tell you you're
forgiven,
Or that it's not necessary to work all the time or that
it's
Been decided that if you lie down no one will die.

If you lie down, no one will die. Isn't that what we are afraid of in our heart of hearts? That if we are not there, something bad will happen and we'll never be able to forgive ourselves? We imagine the worst and create a prison that locks in our body, mind, and spirit. When we don't care for ourselves we are denying the possibility that good things are more likely to be the result than bad ones. When we don't care for ourselves we are doing a disservice to those we love as well as to ourselves. It is important to give yourself the gift of permission. Ultimately that's where loving, honoring, and valuing yourself has to begin.

Things to Think About, Things to Do

When was the last time you did something nice for yourself? When was the last time you took a real vacation?

Have you ever said no to your loved one? Have you ever said no to a medical professional? If not, what would need to happen in order for you to consider it?

Do you now understand the connection between your good health, your energy level, and the quality of care you are able to provide? Since this is the first day of the rest of your life, what realistic new resolution can you make right away to begin to put that understanding into practice?

What can you do to create just a little more balance in your life? What can you do to find just fifteen or twenty minutes of respite every day?

CHAPTER 5

Help Is Not a Dirty Word

Find help as soon as you can. If you refuse help nicely in the beginning, people will never ask you again.

Barb Stutzka, West Concord, MN

Why is it so hard to ask for help? What's a good response to the statement, "Call me if you need me?" How is it that despite the fact we are drowning in responsibility or are really confused about what our next step ought to be, we often respond "no thanks" when help is offered? Where do I find help if I decide I need it, and what can we do about those siblings of ours that just refuse to help out with mom and dad?

Asking for and accepting help is a complex issue. Obviously we first need to recognize that having some help can make a real difference to our loved one's well being and ours as well. Then we need to figure out what we actually need help with and what kind of help we are willing to accept. There are, of course, the practical issues regarding paid help versus friendly help. If this just sounds like more work, another list of things to do, know that it doesn't have to be an overwhelming task but rather just a way to organize thoughts and information you may already have.

Just as with respite, which is designed to give you a relaxing break from your responsibilities, having help can restore your equilibrium because removing some of the responsibility from your shoulders will lessen your stress. It will also enable you to be a more peaceful and effective caregiver because you won't feel so much alone, and that's got to make you a happier and healthier person. It is precisely because you do care that getting some help when you need it is important.

Not all family caregivers need help of course. If your husband is relatively independent despite his disability, or your dad just needs a daily reminder to take his medications, then your caregiving responsibilities may well be very manageable and not an issue of concern at this time. But for those of us that need to help loved ones with personal care on a daily basis, or are part of the sandwich generation caring for elders as well as our own kids, or are just feeling generally overwhelmed by caregiving issues, having help can make a big difference.

The Benefits of Getting Help

1. It can lessen your sense of isolation knowing that other people have an idea of what you are dealing with and are willing to be there for you when needed.
2. It can move the dial on your "worry meter" down to a safe level.
3. It can encourage your loved one to be more independent.
4. It can give you more confidence in your ability to manage your caregiving responsibilities.
5. It can increase your ability to think creatively and expand the options you now have available to you.

To my way of thinking, those are pretty good benefits indeed.

If you can think of some others, write them down on a piece of paper along with the ones I have listed. Stick them on your refrigerator door or some other place where you will see them often. Since asking for help is often such a hard thing to do, we need all the encouragement we can get to do it.

Barriers to Seeking and Accepting Help

The hardest part is fear, i.e., fear of refusal, fear of being misunderstood, or fear that I'll be considered whiny.

E. Dee Manies, Overland Park, KS

Why is seeking and accepting help so darn hard? What prevents us from reaching out or letting others in? I think it has a lot to do with pride because, in addition to helping us recognize our accomplishments and encouraging us to persevere, pride can get in the way of relationships and close us off from others. Pride swells our hearts when our children bring home a report card filled with As, and pride in ourselves is part of the reward for learning a new computer program or losing those five pounds we gained last Christmas. But pride can get in the way when it is the cause of our refusing to apologize to a friend for a hurtful act, or when it won't let us admit we made a bad decision. In the context of caregiving, pride can prolong the time we struggle before we seek assistance, and it can get in the way of accepting help even when it is sincerely offered and very concrete. For men this can be a particular problem since men are supposed to be strong and silent in the face of adversity.

The hardest part about asking for help was shedding the cultural conditioning that men are tough, that men don't cry, that

real men don't each quiche and they should be able to handle
whatever life throws their way.

Ron Perry, Wayne, PA

As Americans we are brought up to be fiercely independent
and, for many of us, very private about our personal lives, too.
Asking for help forces us to admit we can't do everything ourselves and necessitates that we peel away some of the layers
that protect our private lives from public view. These are not
easy things to do. They take time, and doing them often em-
barrasses us. But once we work through our pride, or at least
the portion of it that impacts our willingness to ask for and
receive assistance, our lives and those of our loved ones can be
more enjoyable, less scary, and a great deal safer.

In many circumstances, it isn't only our pride that must be
dealt with. Your husband may be adamant about not wanting
someone else to touch his genitals. Your siblings may repeat-
edly dissuade you from letting others know the true circumstances of your mom's finances. Pride is about self-image. Taking steps that will potentially alter your self-image and also
the image you, your loved one, and your family, project to the
world is a big deal. So much of caregiving occurs behind the
closed doors of bedrooms and bathrooms. No wonder we are
hesitant to ask for help.

We need to understand that there are all sorts of ways that
other people can help without our having to let them see the
most private details of our caregiving. In other cases, of course,
it is help with those personal details that we need the most.
Somewhere along the line we have to strike a balance between
independence and practicality.

Caregiving Is Work

As we become family caregivers, we add work to our already
busy lives. Even though most of us very willingly and lovingly

take on this added responsibility, we must remember that we are doing just that, adding more responsibility and more work. So what happens to all of the other work you were previously doing? Cooking and cleaning and shopping, being a carpool mom for the kids, walking the dog, holding down a job, paying the bills, none of these are going away.

If you can find even one person or one service that can reduce your regular workload by either taking over all or part of one of your regular chores, you'll have more time for your caregiving, and less stress bearing down on you. If you can find a person or service that can help with your specific caregiving responsibilities, you'll be in a better position to meet your non-caregiving responsibilities. Finding help is often difficult for emotional, financial, and geographic reasons, but it can make a big difference in your ability to be an effective caregiver; it can make a big difference in your loved one's well being, and it can make a difference in your own well being and that of other family members as well. It's worth the effort.

Defining the Help You Need

When people offer to help, be ready to give them a date and time when they are needed.

Dick Stone, Oklahoma City, OK

Getting help requires some creativity, and perseverance. You first need to define what you need help with, which tasks or chores would be the easiest to get others to help with, which you really want to do yourself and which if any you can afford to pay others to do. And then, of course, there is the actual reaching out and opening up. You don't need to do it all at once. In fact I wouldn't recommend it. Take it a step at a time so you can get comfortable with the whole idea.

If you are willing to plunge in, defining the help you need

could actually be one of the first things you get help with. What about asking a friend to help you think through your list of responsibilities and put some ideas on paper? If your friend knows you fairly well, perhaps he or she will even begin a list for you. At times that little jumpstart is what it takes, especially if you are like the thirty-eight percent of caregivers who responded in a 1997 survey by the National Alliance for Caregiving and the AARP by saying they didn't know what kind of help would benefit them.

Over the years, I've found a way to think through my own situation for defining the help I need. It does require making lists, at least the first few times you do it, so I wanted to say that up front. But it really isn't an onerous task, and I find it useful to this day. In fact I find when I do make the effort to put things down on paper, rather than just think about them in my head, I have the opportunity to keep the list as a living document that I can add to when I have new thoughts. Inevitably when I go through this process I gain insights that eventually move me to take action, which really is the whole point of making the list in the first place.

A Recipe for Defining and Getting Help

Step 1. Recognize that caregiving, like all jobs, is made up of lots of individual tasks, not all of which are of the same importance. Some tasks take a few minutes, some may take many hours. Some tasks are easy, others require some skill and fortitude. The challenge is to know the difference.

Step 2. Recognize that asking for help is a sign of strength and not of weakness. It means you truly have a grasp on your situation and have come up with a proactive problem-solving technique to try and make things easier or better.

Step 3. Start a list of all your caregiving-related tasks that need to get done in any given week, or at least those you are most concerned about, such as filing insurance forms, arranging your schedule at work so you can meet your obligations there and still be able to take your son to counseling three times a week, getting nutritious meals on the table most nights, lifting, bathing, dressing, and undressing your husband. When you see the types of tasks that are on your list, you'll realize there's a good reason you are so tired and don't have time for yourself.

If this is proving difficult for you, perhaps the following chart will help. It lists some specific needs that many family caregivers have and also some corresponding ways that friends, family, or volunteers could meet those needs.

A Caregiver's List of Needs	How Friends or Family Can Help
A ride to doctor appointments every other Monday	"Chauffeur Service" at a pre-assigned date and time
Getting dinner on the table	A meal prepared and delivered on Tuesdays and Thursdays for the next three months
Dealing with the insurance company	Forms filled out monthly as well as several hours of my time each month to advocate on your behalf
Someone to care about me	A weekly phone call, a shoulder to cry on
Keeping the house clean	A maid brigade every other week, until school starts
Keeping food in the house	Doing the grocery shopping every week for the next two months
Emergency assistance	My commitment to come when you call
Some quiet time alone	Taking your mom out for a ride every other Saturday
Help with household maintenance	A promise to mow your lawn all summer and the availability of my tools and time if we can schedule it in advance

More time	Running weekly errands for you, going to the drugstore, the cleaners, and taking Jake to Sunday school
More money	I can't write you a check but I can go to the discount store and buy you things in bulk
A home care aid	My commitment to coordinate a volunteer team from the church to help out with specific caregiving tasks

Step 4. Clarify your situation using the most distinct categories possible. As you can see, I am a big believer in organizing ideas into categories. It helps me see the big picture and understand how individual activities fit into the puzzle that comprises the caregiving aspects of my life. Categories may include personal care tasks for your loved one, transportation, and household chores. You may think that all your tasks fit neatly into only a few categories, or you may be comfortable with being more specific and thereby have many more categories into which your individual tasks fall. There's no right or wrong. It's all a matter of personal preference.

Step 5. Name your worries. What do you worry about most as a caregiver? Who will help mom if she falls and no one is around? Where will we get the money to pay for John's medications? Who will care for Mary if I get sick? Where can I find affordable daycare? If you are like me, your worries fit into some of the same categories as your tasks, but I think it's important to be able to list your worries specifically. Speaking them out loud or seeing them written on a piece of paper somehow transforms them from abject fears to problems to be solved. That's a more comfortable place for me. It doesn't make my big worries disappear, but at least it lets me approach them in a somewhat rational way. It lets me see them in a different light, and gives me hope that I can find a way to deal with them, rather than being paralyzed into doing nothing until they turn into crises and I am forced to do something.

Step 6. Step back from the edge and assess your options objectively in order to maintain, or regain a sense of calm. This is especially important when you sense things are starting to get a little out of control. I feel so much better after I've gone through this process. It gives me a sense of satisfaction and even relief, as if I've seen a storm coming and I've managed to get home just before the downpour begins. It let's me say that if I try, I just may be able to keep my head above water yet again. It's a calming feeling, one that lets me look at my list of tasks and worries with a less emotional eye and admit which tasks I actually like doing, which I hate or feel incompetent to deal with well, which I really think I have to do myself, at least for the time being, and which are just ho-hum things that have to get done but don't carry any particular emotional impact one way or the other. It helps me think about what tasks I ought to try to get assistance with, which (if any) I can afford to pay someone else to do, or which I might ask a friend or family member, neighbor, or even a volunteer team from the synagogue to help me with.

Perhaps helping your mom with her shower falls into the "I have to do it myself" category, whereas taking her to a regular doctor's appointment is something you can envision someone else doing. Do you enjoy cooking or the time you spend helping your daughter exercise her legs? What can't you stand dealing with or feel insecure about? Is going to the supermarket or managing your brother's medications on your list of things that need to get done but that are no big deal to you? As you are thinking about this, please try and make sure that not everything falls under the " I have to do it myself" category. The idea here is to get a handle on how you can lessen your load, not keep it the same.

Not too long ago I came up with a helpful list; you can find it at the back of this chapter. Making it convinced me that Steven and I really did need to meet with a financial planner. We'd talked about it for a long time, but because the economy had been in such great shape for so long and the stock market was booming, it didn't seem to be a priority. But then the market turned and we began to think we needed some professional advice, especially because retirement issues are looming on the horizon and it is clear to us that Steven will need some personal care services in the future.

Step 7. If you are comfortable doing it, share these thoughts with a close family member, a good friend, another caregiver, or perhaps your clergyman or the employee assistance counselor at work. You might actually want to discuss them with your care recipient if that is possible. The intent here isn't necessarily to get actual physical help or professional advice from this person, but to let you have the benefit of hearing someone else's ideas and insights. Two brains focused on solving a problem are usually more effective than one!

Step 8. As the folks at Nike say, Just Do It! Take a deep breath and actually ask someone to help with one of the tasks on your list, or ask for guidance in resolving your most persistent worry. I'd suggest starting with something small, especially if you are looking for hands-on assistance or something that requires someone doing you a favor. You may have to ask for help a few times before you begin to get comfortable with the whole idea. With practice, it really does get easier. Just one more bit of advice on this score, I promise: Don't forget to be open to those offering to help. With your list of tasks in hand and your sense of your priorities and concerns, you'll be better able to take advantage of opportunity when it knocks. You'll have a ready response when someone says, "Call me if you need me." You'll be able to say, "I would really like to find a pharmacy that delivers, but I just haven't had the time to do the research, would you be willing to do it for me?"

Help Caŋ Coɱe iŋ Maŋy Guises

The kind of help that I need the most these days is assistance with household maintenance issues. I can handle Steven's care needs. Because we've been doing it for so long now our morning routine of showering together and my dressing him as I'm getting dressed seems normal, at least for us. When I travel we obviously have to have a home care aide sleep over and attend to morning and evening necessities.

But keeping the house in good shape is another story. I enjoy cooking, and can certainly handle the laundry and some other basic household chores, but I am not handy when it comes to fix-it things. I don't really enjoy gardening, and quite frankly I don't have the time, given the fact that I have prioritized meeting Steven's care needs myself, putting a lot of my energy into NFCA, keeping an eye on my own health and having some time to spend with our granddaughter. We certainly aren't rich, but right now we can afford to have someone mow the lawn, clean the house, and keep the gutters clear. Steven and I have agreed we will continue to pay for those services as long as we can.

But there is some help that no amount of money can buy. It's the help I need when Steven falls during a transfer, especially when it's a transfer from toilet to wheelchair and he ends up on the cold tile floor caught between the wall and the wheelchair in our postage stamp size bathroom. It's real time emergency help I need then, and it necessitates that I rely on others. That's when I give Allen or Tony a call.

Allen is one of our neighbors. He lives directly across the street. He's tall, well over six feet, and solid. Somehow, miraculously it seems to me, Allen is usually available when I need his help. Despite a busy travel schedule, he's at home more often than not when I call. I've come to think of Allen as my white knight who comes over at a moment's notice and, with a few deft strokes, manages to pick Steven up and right him in his wheelchair. It's such a comfort knowing that Allen lives across the street and is so willing to lend a hand.

It took a lot for us to get over the shame and the embarrassment of having to ask for help in such personal circumstances, and we didn't do it easily. I recall one time when Steven fell and we were still trying to deal with such situations on our own. I used a sheet to drag him from the bathroom, across the wooden floor and down the hall, past the guest room and his office, and then onto the carpeting in the master bedroom.

There was no place at all in the bathroom that he could hold on to and from which I could try to bend his legs and position them in such a way that, working together, we could maneuver him into a standing position. At least in our bedroom there was a bed frame with decorative cutouts that work well as hand holds. First I had to get Steven's body in a straight line so that I could get the sheet under him sufficiently enough that it would carry him along as I dragged it, huffing and puffing, toward the bedroom. It required strength I really didn't have.

Once in the bedroom we struggled and struggled some more until we could control the spasticity in his legs and get his knees bent and enough of his upper body on the bed so that finally I could lift his lower body and legs onto the bed. From there we were able to transfer him back into the wheelchair, as we did each morning. The whole process took about forty-five exhausting minutes to go a distance of just twenty-three feet. Steven's skin was rubbed raw and my back was pretty sore. That was it. We weren't going to try that ever again. Reality was pushing pride aside. We agreed we needed to reach out to neighbors, and that's what we started to do.

I'm actually very lucky. If Allen isn't home, I know I can always turn to Tony who lives next door. Tony isn't quite as tall as Allen, but he is younger and very strong, and most importantly, always willing to help at a moment's notice.

Steven had bladder surgery this past spring. In the scheme of things it was a relatively minor operation, but given his disability it totally destroyed whatever strength he had to help himself, especially because there was now a row of stitches across his abdomen. Bending from the waist was particularly painful and there was no way we could get him in and out of bed each morning and night using our usual transfer technique. Insurance wasn't willing to pay for home care assistance so we had to find help on our own.

The first night Steven was home from the hospital I asked Tony if he would be willing to come over and help me get Steven into bed. "Of course I'll come. What time?" he said. He came that night at 10:15 and the next morning at 6:30, and he continued to come morning and night for the next five days, until we felt comfortable doing the transfer on our own. He made me promise I wouldn't hesitate to call if we needed his help again. He was embarrassed when I kept telling him how grateful I was. "Don't think about it. That's what neighbors are for. I'm glad to help, really," he said. And I knew he meant it.

I recall one Sunday afternoon when Steven had slipped out of his wheelchair during a transfer (we seemed to go through a period of several months before we had come to terms with the fact that the stair glide we had installed to get Steven from house to garage and back again was no longer working for us, and we were experiencing the consequences) and neither Allen nor Tony was at home. Unfortunately, neither was Kathy, whom I've also called on from time to time. It seemed we were the only ones around on that lovely sunny Sunday. Bereft of neighbors, or at least those I felt comfortable enough asking at the time, I called the fire department. If people ask them to get cats out of trees, I surmised, they can surely help lift a man off of the floor. Sure enough, three members of the rescue squad showed up within fifteen minutes. "Any time ma'am," they said with a smile.

I've become very good at asking for help, at putting necessity first and pride last. I've learned that caregiving is more than a one-person job and that you need to know when something is beyond your capabilities. I've learned how absolutely critical it is to make a conscious effort to put a network of support in place, to have people you can call on in an emergency. I've also learned it doesn't just happen. It requires an effort and a breaking down of barriers. You have to let people into your life, to tell your story, to let them see your vulnerability as well as your strength. It's the price we have to pay, but the rewards are well worth it.

We didn't know that Allen lived across the street when we bought our house, or that Tony would move in next door, but as Steven has become increasingly disabled, we have come to realize how critical it is to establish a core group of people that we can rely on. Allen and his wife Alice recently put their house up for sale. I waited anxiously to find out who our new neighbors would be. When the "under contract" sign went up in their yard, I called Alice. After asking the obvious curiosity questions "Do they have kids? What line of work are they in?" I asked the ones that were most important to me. "Is the husband tall, well built? Does he seem the sort to be willing to be part of our care team?" Alice was able to answer my first two questions. "I think they are in their late twenties, maybe early thirties. He is fairly tall," she said, "but maybe not as tall as Allen."

I'll have to wait to get the answer to my third question. The new neighbors have not yet moved in. But when they do I'll go over and introduce myself. Of course I won't pop the question right away. I want to establish a relationship first, make sure we are going to enjoy being each other's neighbors, but after we've gotten to know each other a bit, I won't hesitate. Knowing where my emergency support is coming from is just too important.

Thoughts on Where to Look for Help

The person who says "I have two hours on Friday afternoon or Saturday morning . . . could I pick up your children and take them to the park?" or "I would love to come on Thursday and bring dinner, if you would like". . . . These folks are angels in disguise."

K. Metzguer, Hillsborough, NC

The number of things family caregivers need help with is seemingly endless. There is no one solution that is right for everyone. Where you live may well be a factor, as may your income, too high for government programs, too low to allow you to pay for services. Nevertheless, here are some possible directions.

Perhaps there are county services such as Meals on Wheels that can bring nourishing food to your dad every day, so that you don't have to drive over there as often. Perhaps you can rearrange your work schedule so that you can have half a day off every Friday afternoon during which to deal with your sister's appointments and insurance paperwork. Is there a parish nurse service available through your church?

Can you afford to hire a home care aide for several hours a week to give your partner a bed bath? Will your best friend's teenage son mow your lawn in the summer and shovel the snow from your driveway in the winter? If you live in Los Angeles and your parents live in Omaha can you find a geriatric care manager there to assess your parents' situation and provide you with weekly reports? Might a nursing student be willing to watch your disabled child once a week so you can more easily run errands?

Will your brother agree to help finance your mom's care, if you agree to be the primary caregiver? Will your neighbors agree to pitch in and bring over meals four times a week so you don't have to think about what's for dinner? I asked some longstanding caregivers for their advice on where to find help. Here's what they said.

Begin by finding out what is available from the health insurance company, Medicare or Medicaid. Then check with state programs, community services and church programs in your community. . . . With planning and organization you can work toward having the help you need.

Linda. Reid, Oneonta, AL

I've asked at the local privately owned drug store, asked neighbors, asked nurses at my husband's dialysis clinic. . . .

Paulette. Miley, Chesnee, SC

When I saw what was coming, I immediately increased our world and put us in a position to meet more people. Mainly church groups, etc.

Jeannine Tjugum, Hartland, WI

In the Resource Section of this book I list a variety of organizations including their national phone numbers and Web site addresses, but it is important to remember that ultimately the resources you are most likely to need are local. The purpose of giving you these national contacts is so that you will have a starting point from which to begin your search.

A Cautionary Note

I wish I could say that making lists, and knowing people and places to reach out to guarantees that you will definitely get help, but unfortunately that isn't the case. What it does do though is put you in a much better position to get assistance than you would have been in if you hadn't gone through the process. But it is important to be realistic. There will definitely be disappointments.

People are very kind, but they will not show up. They are busy; they are sick, they are over-committed. Probably they are scared to see him being so disabled.

Lori Brown, Richmond, CA

*The hardest part is not getting it [help] after finally working up
the nerve to ask for it.*

Susan Kiser Scarff, Phonenix, AZ

All in the Family

If you have family members who help you out with your caregiving responsibilities, you are very fortunate. Helping each
other can bring close families even closer. In families where
there traditionally have been tensions, it can help ease those
tensions. And in families that haven't been particularly close,
it can be the catalyst that helps build strong bonds.

Steven and I are lucky in that regard; our daughter Darryn
and son-in-law Steve (note the use of the nickname, that's how
we distinguish between the two) moved from North Carolina
to Maryland a few years ago. They bought a house just ten
minutes from ours. Darryn is often available to help out if I
have a dinner meeting downtown or some other engagement
that throws off my set schedule. She'll stop by on her way
home from work after picking my granddaughter Kaylyn up
from daycare and get Steven his dinner, which I have ready in
the fridge. She just needs to heat it up in the microwave, set
the table, and get him a glass of juice. Steven has the pleasure
of seeing his daughter and granddaughter, and I have the piece
of mind that comes from knowing things are under control.

Darryn often asks me to help her out as well, and I like that.
It makes ours a symbiotic relationship. We help each other.
Sometimes she'll ask me to stop by her house at lunchtime
and let the dog in if it looks like it will rain, and sometimes
she asks me to baby sit, which of course I love to do.

If your family doesn't help out, realize that you are not
alone. According to the National Association of Geriatric Care

Managers in Tucson, in 99.9 percent of cases there is one sibling that takes on most of the responsibility of caring for mom or dad. This can range from being the prime decision-maker to the major hands-on caregiver.

Spousal caregivers and parents with special needs kids are often going it alone too. In some situations spousal caregivers don't want to let their children know how difficult things are. I often hear, "They have their own families to worry about. I couldn't possibly ask them for help. I don't want to burden them with my problems." Parents of special needs children generally get more help from family members than do other types of caregivers, but it often peters out as the child gets older and is often non-existent when the child becomes an adult.

The reasons for this are as complicated as the family dynamics involved. Some families are close and have always reached out to each other. Others are barely on speaking terms. Siblings have rivalries. Adult children are estranged. Parents are divorced. And then of course there are those of us who think we shouldn't have to ask family. Family members ought to recognize that we need help and offer it.

My brothers and sister helped out when they could, but even though I was feeling totally desperate, I felt that I should not be asking for help and did not share how bad things had gotten.

Melissa McKerrow, Rockville, MD

A Family Meeting

Getting family members to help you is not an impossible task. It isn't fair, though, to think that everyone can read your mind, especially if they live far away and don't see what is actually involved. That's why professionals often say the most important thing to do is have a family meeting, and do it as early in the caregiving process as possible. This will allow everyone to understand the situation and what is likely to happen in the future.

Having the meeting in person is of course ideal, but if that is totally impossible consider telephone conferencing. If everyone is on-line, then e-mail, instant messaging, or a private chat room are alternatives, but having the meeting in person really is best. You can see each other's facial expressions and body language. Making an effort to get to the meeting place shows a commitment to at least taking a real look at the issues, and it can be an opportunity for family members who haven't been together in a while to reunite around a common concern. If done early, it can preclude one person unwittingly having to carry the bulk of the caregiving alone. If you are already that bulk-carrying caregiver, the meeting is a mechanism to help you lighten your load.

You'll need to decide whether or not the care recipient should be present. That will depend upon their state of mind and whether or not they are resistant to having help. The advantage to having everyone at the meeting is that you are all involved and can have your say. The meeting is not supposed to lead to a family conspiracy against the person that needs care. Its goal is exactly the opposite, to bring you all closer together and come up with a sound plan for helping you and managing the care of your loved one. If having a family meeting sounds like an idea you'd like to try, here are some tips to keep in mind.

1. Plan ahead. Give yourself time to prepare. Suggest several alternate dates.
2. Have a facilitator at the meeting, especially if you think the meeting is likely to be divisive. A trusted member of the clergy, a social worker, geriatric care manager, or nurse who is familiar with your care recipient's condi-

tion are all good choices. That person can keep the conversation on track, referee if voices are raised, provide an impartial point of view, and share information about your loved one's illness, the realities of insurance coverage and long-term care financing. They can also touch on the mounting emotional stress of caregiving that everyone will have to deal with as time goes by.

3. At the meeting it is perfectly okay to have a written list in front of you outlining key points you want to make. It won't ruin your credibility. On the contrary, it will show that you've thought this through carefully.

4. When describing your situation, be as specific as possible. Try drawing a verbal picture of a typical day. Use imagery and statistics to make your points memorable.

5. Get feedback. If people aren't offering any, the facilitator's job is to stir conversation. If there is no facilitator involved, then you'll have to take the lead by saying, "I'd like to know what you're thinking or feeling." Don't be surprised if some people are in denial and others are nervous or defensive. People need time to absorb all you've said, but they should be reminded that if something happened to you, someone else would have to step in. Better to preclude that from happening by working out a shared caring plan now.

6. It's good to add a little levity to the situation. Humorous anecdotes and jokes can break the tension and preserve everyone's dignity. The facilitator can both initiate this and draw the group back to the discussion at hand.

7. At the end of the meeting it is important to have closure. What has been decided? Will there be another meeting, if so who is in charge of arranging it? As the organizer of the first meeting you should send out a memo listing the key points of the discussion and next steps. Agree to stay in touch by whatever means are most practical. You've started a dialogue. It is important to keep it going.

8. End with a pizza or some other prepared meal. Sitting around the table together is a good reminder that this was a family meeting, not a business one. If time and energy allow, perhaps some of the help can begin that very day, with Nancy gathering up the insurance policies to review, and Dave raking the leaves from the lawn.

An Asking for Help Success Story

Sue Tissian is a caregiver for her husband Sam who had a stroke some years ago. She hadn't told anyone about how she felt about her changed life until she decided to respond to an NFCA request for caregivers to share their stories and a list of needs and wishes that would make their caregiving situation better.

Something inside her told Sue it was time to take a look at her concerns. She sat down and wrote her story—just five short paragraphs and a needs/wish list of only four items. It wasn't easy to do, she told us. It brought a lot of emotions to the surface and it made her admit how difficult it was to be a family caregiver. Once it was done, however, she felt better, and so decided to show it to her daughter Marlene. This is what Sue Tissian wrote.

I am a 73 year old healthy woman, caring for my 74 year old spouse. Though I have some physical problems of my own, they take a back seat to the needs of my husband, Sam. His stroke left him with a right side weakness, which requires him to use a walker, and severe aphasia and apraxia. (Aphasia is the loss or impairment of the power to use words. Apraxia is the inability to execute complex coordinated movements). Though he uses Metro Access for his weekly speech therapy sessions, I drive him to wherever his needs take us. I now manage all household, financial, physical, and communication needs for both of us.

I feel overwhelmed most of the time and accomplish very little except meeting our immediate needs. He does not require constant care. He is capable of caring for himself almost completely so I can leave him for long periods, but I feel guilty whenever I do.

Another difficult adjustment for me is the autonomous decision-making. This is no longer a shared responsibility; it has become a very heavy burden.

We would like to move to more accessible living quarters because I can no longer maintain the grounds and repairs on this aging house, but the thought of getting rid of 48 years of accumulated junk puts me in a state of immobility.

After over 50 years of marriage, I find that I am not the strong burden carrier I always thought I was. I miss our conversations, our spontaneous activities, and our independence.

If I had a dream list, it would include some of the following:

1. The sale of our house.
2. Finding and moving to a new home.
3. Traveling again, whenever the desire arose.
4. Another regular exercise program that he would enjoy.

As soon as Marlene read her mom's story, she and her husband Barry leapt into action. They hired a realtor, and within six weeks, Sue's home had been sold and a new home in a well-run retirement community had been found. Marlene and Barry took care of all the details. Sue's job was to make the final decisions and sign the papers.

I had no idea about the depth of mom's anguish or that the reason she hadn't sold the house was because she perceived it to be an enormous task to move. Whenever we were together she was in good spirits. She seemed to be coping with whatever things life threw at her. I wish I would have known just how important it was for her to move. Selling the house was not a difficult task for us to take care of. I'm just glad she finally shared her story with us.

Sue later said this:

. . . I kept telling myself that my kids have their own lives to live. I don't want to burden them with my problems. Little did I know how much they wanted to help. I can't believe how relieved I am now, how much happier.

Suzanne's List of Major Tasks, Attitudes, and Worries

Tasks	Attitudes Like (L) Dislike/No Time (DL/NT) Must Do Myself (MDM) Ho-Hum (HH)	Worries
Steven's Personal Care—List A		
Transfers—morning, evening, when going out, in bathroom	MDM for now	Is our emergency network of neighbors large enough so that we don't wear out our welcome if Steven should need help on a regular basis for a while, i.e., as he did getting in and out of bed after he had bladder surgery?
All ADLS—Transfers, showering, dressing, toileting, catheterizing, eating, medication management, coordinating our mutual bedtime	MDM for now	Applies to all ADL tasks: How do I make things as tolerable for Steven as possible when I'm traveling?
Household Chores—List B		
Cooking	L	
Food shopping	L	
Laundry	HH	
Housework	DL/NT	What are our options if/when we can no longer afford to pay for these services—will we have to move?
Gardening/lawn Maintenance	DL/NT	Same as above
House Maintenance	DL/NT	Same as above
Finances—List C		
Pay our regular bills	HH	It's not a problem now, but Steven will most likely retire in a year or so.
Banking	HH	
Getting medications and medical supplies	HH	Now we have a good pharmacy plan and our insurance covers most of the homecare equipment and supplies we need. This won't be the case under Medicare, unless things change.
Filing insurance claims	DL/NT—I really hate filling out forms.	Now we only have to file forms for PT services. Will there be a time when we have lots of forms to fill out.
Financial Planning	Not a question of like or dislike. I know it is something that must be done in a more detailed way than we have in the past	What are our options if/when we can no longer afford to pay for the services that allow us to stay in the house, or living here just becomes impractical? Will we be able to pay for home care services when Steven needs them on a regular basis? What if a nursing home is inevitable? What about me—will we have the funds to pay for my homecare when I need it.

CHAPTER 6

Beyond You and Me

Throughout this book I have been talking about the personal side of caregiving, how it affects our emotions, our relationships, our activities, and our physical health. But I haven't really said anything yet about the public side of caregiving. "Public side," you might be asking, "what public side? Caregiving is something that happens within a family." And you'd be right. Caregiving is something that happens within a family, but it also exists outside of and beyond the family.

In this day and age, caregiving is a social issue. It is of concern to policy makers and politicians at the federal, state, and local levels, to employers, insurers, and healthcare providers. It is a topic of discussion in faith communities and the subject of research in universities. Today caregiving is much more than a personal family issue. It is the issue of our age because it will sooner or later affect every family in America, and we are not prepared either as individuals or as a society to deal with it.

Then and Now

Of course families have always taken care of their ill or disabled loved ones. Neighbors helped neighbors if they didn't have family around, and even communities helped care for the ill among them, but the nature of caregiving has changed radically. In the past—

- Families didn't provide care for as many years as we do now.
- Families didn't care for loved ones who were as ill, aged, or disabled as ours.
- Families didn't live in as highly mobile a society as we do.
- Families didn't care for loved ones when so many women were employed and waited until their thirties or even early forties to have children.
- Families didn't provide care at a time when healthcare costs and the question of who should pay for them were issues of such concern.
- Families didn't provide care at a time when medical science had unlocked secrets about how to save and extend lives in ways that were previously unimaginable.
- Families didn't care for loved ones at a time when the average age of the population was on the rise and aging baby boomers would soon be entering their senior years.

It is for all these reasons that caregiving is so very different today than it ever was before. It is because of all these changes, which have occurred in a relatively short period of time, that the word *caregiver* even exists. The first recorded use of it was only in 1975, according to Merriam-Webster's Collegiate Dictionary. The term *family caregiver* still hasn't made it into the tenth edition of that dictionary, and it was just published in 2001.

I don't know about you, but I find it rather disconcerting that we family caregivers don't even exist as far as the arbiters of American English are concerned, despite the fact that over fifty million people a year provide some level of care to an ill, aged, or disabled family member. References to family doctors go back as far as 1846 and the relatively new term, *family practice*, sometimes referred to as *family medicine*, showed up in 1969.

It makes me very sad that nobody really cares about the caregivers.

Joan Smith, Revere, PA

If you are shaking your head and asking, "why is she trying to politicize what for me is a very personal undertaking," please bear with me. There may well be some of you who are still uncomfortable with thinking of yourself as a family caregiver, even after reading this book, and some of you may find the whole idea of family caregivers as a specific subset of the population a disturbing one. But that's exactly why I want to share with you some of what I have learned over the past ten years, about how much things have changed in terms of health and healthcare during the past century, and how it is having a very real daily effect on me and my family and on you and yours.

Healthcare Achievements 1900–2001

All across this country, public personalities and unknown citizens, both young and old, are alive today and have a meaningful quality of life because of the extraordinary advances that have occurred in medical science and technology during the twentieth century.

Christopher Reeve played Superman in the movies, the man of steel able to leap tall buildings at a single bound. The irony of course is that since the horseback riding accident in 1995 that left him a quadriplegic, Christopher Reeve has truly become a superman, a man with an inner strength of steel that supports the heady pace he pursues as a spokesperson and fundraiser for spinal chord injury research. If Chris's accident had occurred five years earlier the medical knowledge, skills, and equipment needed to save and maintain his life most likely would not have been available.

Also in 1995, on September 15th, Kaylee Davis was born with a rare genetic disorder called Camptomelic Displasia. She has heart, lung, orthopedic and hearing problems, to name just a few. She requires twelve medications a day in order to survive, and they must be administered via a "G" tube that goes directly into her stomach, as does the liquid food that comprises her diet. She has had more operations in her short life than most of us will ever have in our lifetime. Kaylee's home was a hospital's intensive care unit until she was five weeks old. Without the advances in medical science that have occurred in the past six years, Kaylee would not be alive today. In fact, doctors gave her little chance of surviving, since most children with her condition die at birth. Lest you think Kaylee's life is only about medical interventions, let me assure you that she is a bright and perky little girl who knows how to have fun and is as cute as can be. Her three older siblings dote on her.

Given the medical wonders of our time it is easy to forget that in the early nineteen hundreds infectious diseases were the most common cause of death. More than 675,000 people died from the influenza outbreak of 1918, just in the United States. Although it is commonplace today, penicillin was the new miracle drug of the early 1940s. A vaccine for polio, the great crippler of children, became available in 1955. This was soon followed by an oral vaccine in 1963 that was much easier to administer and therefore became accessible to an even larger number of people.

Everyone from my baby boom generation has a smallpox mark somewhere on their upper arm, a sign that we had been vaccinated against this disfiguring and deadly disease. Everyone from Generation X, including my daughter, has one too. But not my granddaughter. In the late 1970s the United States Public Health Service advised against inoculating children for smallpox because it was no longer seen as a threat to the American public. We had for all intents and purposes wiped out one of the most infectious diseases in the world.

It was only in 1978 that the first sign of what would later be called AIDS showed up in the United States. It shortly became an epidemic and was considered a terminal disease. Although many people still die from AIDS, it has been reclassified from a terminal to a chronic disease because of the many drugs that have been developed in just this short period of time to keep the AIDS-causing virus under control.

One of history's most extraordinary scientific efforts, the charting of the human genome, was begun in 1990. Completion was scheduled for 2005 but by June 2000 a working draft had already been produced and final completion is now set for 2003. These sorts of rapid discoveries are changing the face of medicine almost on a daily basis. Who ever heard of stem cell research even a few years ago? Cloning used to belong to the realm of science fiction, but no more. Today it is the subject of a very real ethical debate.

If you drew a chart of all the scientific and medical advances since 1900, you would see what is often referred to as a "J curve," one that very slowly starts to move, almost laterally at first, and then shoots rapidly and radically upward. Such change in one aspect of our lives has a direct effect on other aspects as well, but that doesn't mean these changes are absorbed and integrated into society at the same breathtaking speed. In fact social change always occurs a great deal more slowly.

The Snail's Pace of Social Change

Although we have learned how to save the lives of people who are injured by gunfire or who suffer a heart attack, we haven't put in place an organized, affordable, and easy-to-access way for them to learn about and obtain the necessary services and social supports they need to continue having meaningful lives. Once that survivor leaves the hospital it is up to her and her family to figure out how they will put bread on the table, pay bills, move easily around the community, and continue to have a network of friends and family willing to help out during a crisis and long into the future.

Doctors can restore a man to functional health after a stroke, but there is no guarantee that he and his wife will be able to cope with the fact that he can no longer speak nor walk as steadily as he did before, and there is no one person, or team of people, for them to call who will guide them when they need help navigating the new and rocky terrain of their daily life.

One of the things that frustrates caregivers more than others is the fact that they are left on their own to wade through a choppy sea of disparate programs that may or may not be open to them or meet their needs. Everyone working in the field of caregiving agrees our system of social supports is hopelessly fragmented and insufficient, and there is no good and easy way to fix it. Caregivers need the mental acuity and passionate perseverance of a Sherlock Holmes to solve even one part of their support-needs puzzle.

Christopher Reeve and Kaylee Davis can truly be called miracles of modern medicine, but it takes the hard work, the constant vigilance, and the enduring love of their families to ensure that their lives have quality as well as years. Science and medicine may be on a J curve, a rocket-powered trip of discovery, but the path to implementing the day-to-day rights and services needed by the Christopher Reeves and Kaylee Davises of this world is traveled by well-meaning and dedicated people riding ox carts to reach their destination. This vast difference in the speed of change between science and society is one of the primary reasons that caregiving is, and will continue to be, such a challenge for both caregivers and care receivers unless something can be done to bring them closer together.

The Aging of the Population

One of the outcomes of all of these scientific and medical discoveries is that most of us are living longer and healthier lives. My mother turned eighty-five-years old in March 2002. She's in good health for her age and leads an active life as a volunteer, student, grandmother, and great-grandmother. She is constantly amazed that she is still alive because both of her parents died at what we would today consider to be quite young ages, her father at fifty-eight and her mother at sixty-seven. They both died from heart attacks, suddenly and unexpectedly. Given the fact that they were born in the late 1800s that's not surprising. Both of my maternal grandparents actually beat the odds. The average life span in 1900 was only forty-seven. Today it is seventy-six.

By the time I was thirteen, all four of my grandparents had died. But my mother has already lived to see her grandchildren married and become parents themselves. One of my favorite photographs is of me, my mom, my daughter, and her daughter—four generations all alive at the same time. In 1900 only twenty-five percent of newborns had four living grandparents. Sixty-six percent did in 2001.

My mom is part of the fastest growing age cohort in the country. Today there are four million people in the United States eighty-five or older and by 2050 there are expected to be nineteen million, but at the beginning of the twentieth century there were only about 1,000 people who reached that advanced age. Demographers project that by 2030 there will be more than 380,000 people that are at least 100 years old. Some of you may well be among them.

Because so many people are living longer, even the definition of old has changed. Researchers now divide the sixty-five-plus population into three segments. There are the "young-old" (sixty-five to seventy), the "old" (seventy-five to eighty-four), and the "oldest-old" (eighty-five plus).

We truly live in an age that is radically different from previous ones, and because of that the role we are playing as family caregivers is new, too. As we have seen there are both positive and negative consequences to the amazing scientific and medical achievements that occurred in the twentieth century. There are more developmentally delayed children alive today than ever before because medical science has learned how to save preemie babies; I find this to be a particularly painful example of the disconnect between medicine and real life.

Quicker and Sicker

Given the advances in medical science it is not surprising that the practice of medicine has changed over the years, and it is not surprising that the costs have gone up as well. Just think about the alphabet of high-tech medical tests that have become so familiar to us, EKG, CAT Scan, MRI. Managed care seemed to fall into our lives out of nowhere as an answer to the rising costs of care. It sounded great in theory but the fact that many HMOs are quitting Medicare and that consumers who have a choice are opting more and more for preferred provider programs suggests that medicine needs to be high quality and consumer friendly as well as cost effective.

The healthcare we knew in our youth is definitely a thing of the past. When laws have to be passed to ensure that women can stay in the hospital for twenty-four hours after they deliver a baby, something is definitely out of whack. If you or your loved one have had cause to be in the hospital recently, you know that the maternity ward isn't the only place that is on a fast track in-and-out schedule. Hospital stays are getting shorter all the time. There is even a term for this quickening pace of discharge. It is referred to as "quicker and sicker."

This of course is no laughing matter. Just because people are being sent home sooner doesn't mean that they are healing any faster than they did before; it's just that the place where healing occurs has shifted from hospital to home. And that of course is where family caregivers come in. Families are being asked to do for their loved ones what a team of healthcare workers used to do in the hospital.

Some family caregivers have to monitor the intravenous flow of medications that could only have been provided in a hospital setting just a few years ago. Others must learn how to clean and dress serious open wounds that only nurses or doctors were allowed to treat in the past. Feeding tubes, ventilators, catheters, and syringes—you name it—family caregivers are becoming all too familiar with medical equipment and jargon. On the one hand we are being thrust into the role of healthcare provider. On the other we are rarely provided the solid training we need to feel comfortable and competent in this role. We learn by trial and error, not on a dummy in a classroom setting under the watchful eye of a professor, but in our own homes on someone we love.

This just doesn't make sense. Doctors don't treat their family members precisely because of the emotional connection. They go through twelve years of education and training before they are considered sufficiently qualified in their area of specialization to be given full responsibility for a severely ill patient. Nurses have years of training and must pass a rigorous exam and work in a clinical setting before they are allowed to put RN after their name. Physical and occupational therapists are certified. Nursing assistants are required by federal law to have at least seventy-five hours of training and take an exam before they are certified to work with patients.

Not so for family caregivers. In a series of focus groups held by the United Hospital Fund of New York in 1997, family caregivers talked about how they experienced the hospital discharge process. Their comments were integrated into a groundbreaking report, *Rough Crossings: Family Caregivers' Odysseys through the Health Care System.*

Caregivers experienced discharge from the hospital as an abrupt, upsetting event because hospital staff failed to prepare them technically and emotionally for changes in the patient's condition. In many cases, participants reported, the patient after discharge required nursing skills or equipment they did not possess and had little time to acquire.

One caregiver whose husband had had a stroke talked about her concerns regarding the use of a feeding tube with confusing computer settings that she was expected to monitor.

> I was terrified of it . . . It's broken twice. When we left the hospital they showed me 1,2,3, and that's it. They said, "Don't worry, you'll learn it."

A man whose wife had MS and underwent surgery for a leg infection thought that at the time of discharge his wife would be in the same shape she had been in upon entering the hospital. He was not told that she was incontinent or that her bandages would need changing. During the first night home when her bandages were oozing and the bed was wet with urine he found out. "I didn't know what to do, who to call, or who to get angry at" he said in total frustration.

These are not isolated statements. In NFCA's 2001 survey of self-identified family caregivers half of the respondents said they had not been given the training they needed. They had to figure things out on their own.

The Two Different Worlds of Chronic Care and Acute Care

One of the main reasons that all of these outlandish situations exist is because the ways we finance, deliver, and provide healthcare in America are antithetical to the kind of care that the majority of people need. Our entire healthcare system has always been built on an acute care model and not a chronic care model, or even a combination of the two. Acute care deals with here-and-now problems that require immediate attention—an appendix that needs to come out, a car accident victim who must be operated on immediately in order to stop internal bleeding. In acute care medicine, cure is always the goal.

In chronic care situations, the kind that caregivers deal with every day, cure is not possible. Chronic care situations are long-term and are not only medical in nature. They cross the line and require functional assistance, such as transportation and personal care. There are psychosocial and environmental issues that must be dealt with, such as the need to build a new self-image after an amputation or figuring out how to make your home wheelchair accessible. The treatment of chronic conditions requires a holistic approach to healthcare, but unfortunately, American doctors are not trained to treat chronic conditions or to teach patients and their families how to manage them. This is a growing problem because care of the chronically ill accounts for more than seventy-seven percent of all healthcare expenditures.

It is not only the training of doctors that creates this disconnect between what patients and families need and what healthcare provides. Physicians aren't paid to provide the kind of care needed by the chronically ill. Listen to this testimony given by Dr. Alan Lazaroff, Director of Geriatric Medicine and a specialist in chronic illness care at the Centura Health system in Colorado.

> Much of my most important work is unrecognized and uncompensated— adjustment of medication, early detection of problems, referrals to and coordination of other services, teaching and counseling. If I hospitalize a patient, I can bill Medicare every day I make a hospital visit, never mind whether this is the most appropriate treatment. If I meet with family members of a patient with Alzheimer's disease, coordinate with other professionals, counsel patients and families about both the benefits and limitations of aggressive treatment, and help my patients cope with the emotional consequences of their illness, I can bill nothing.

It's clear that American healthcare is out of sync with the reality of life in America today, a reality in which chronic illnesses and family caregiving have the starring roles.

Healthcare Insurance, Public and Private

Medicare and Medicaid are the government's two major healthcare financing programs. Medicare is America's answer to healthcare financing for the elderly, and Medicaid was developed to pay for healthcare services for the poor and disabled. Not everyone is on Medicare or Medicaid, of course, but private insurers often take their cues from what Medicare does and does not cover, so the Medicare rules have relevance for all of us. So do the Medicaid rules, because those of us who have a loved one in need of nursing home care usually have to decide whether to apply for Medicaid, a decision that has significant financial and emotional consequences.

Medicare

Medicare was instituted with much fanfare in the 1960s. It was designed to pay for hospital care and doctors' visits and it was aimed at a senior population that, for the most part, was in its sixties and needed treatment for immediate acute care problems of short duration, conditions such as a broken hip or pneumonia. But as we've seen, a great deal has happened since then. A great many of the folks who were in their mid fifties and mid sixties when the program began are in their eighties and nineties today. They are suffering from chronic conditions, such as Alzheimer's disease and other dementias, Parkinson's disease, diabetes, emphysema, long-term cancers, and the aftermath of a stroke, which they were much less likely to survive in the 1960s. In fact today, over 100 million people in America are living with at least one chronic condition.

The kind of care today's old and oldest-old seniors need now is more extensive than the care they needed thirty years ago. It is more long term, and much of it isn't quite medical, although it is necessitated by medical conditions or the frailties that come with old age. Some need help maintaining a household, including shopping, paying bills, and housekeeping. Others can't manage these tasks and also are unable to take care of their personal care needs, such as dressing, toileting, bathing, and other activities of daily living. Between ages sixty-five and sixty-nine only nine percent of the population requires such help, but within the eighty-five-plus population fifty percent of individuals need such assistance.

Medicare was never designed to pay for the long-term personal care and therapeutic services that people with chronic conditions need. They just aren't part of the Medicare package. In fact Medicare doesn't even talk about personal care. It inappropriately, and I think pejoratively, refers to the type of services provided by family caregivers as "custodial care," and as you and I know, what we do is far more than watch over our loved ones, which is how the dictionary defines the word custodial. But regardless of what words you use to describe the services family caregivers provide, many people just assume that Medicare covers them, and therefore they and their families have a rude awakening when they least expect it. And, as we all do know, Medicare doesn't pay for all those prescription drugs that are a major part of today's medical treatment regimen, and that is why Congress has been struggling with how to help seniors cover the extraordinary cost of medicines.

Geez, the things we do for no pay; the things we can't get because Medicare won't cover them.

Paulette Miley, Chesnee, SC

In addition, Medicare functions under a whole list of quirky rules that make it difficult even for people who would seem to be eligible for services to actually obtain them. One such example is the "homebound rule" that applies to Medicare home health services. Medicare will pay for home healthcare services including personal care if they are prescribed by a doctor, and are directly related to a specific medical condition, such as a hip replacement or the need for a feeding tube. Under the "homebound rule" however, patients are virtual prisoners in their own home. Absences must be "infrequent" and "of short duration" or for medical treatment. That means no going out for a pizza or even to a funeral. In the summer of 2002, due to the efforts of David Jayne, an ALS sufferer, the regulations were clarified to explain that going to adult daycare or a movie were examples of infrequent activities of short duration that should not disqualify patients from receiving Medicare home health benefits. Seems crazy that we need advocacy to allow our loved ones to go out doors, but when it comes to Medicare that is indeed the case.

Medicaid

Unlike Medicare, Medicaid does pay for some long-term care services for people meeting its strict financial guidelines. These services vary from state to state, but the vast majority pay the cost of care in a nursing home or other institutional setting. The law has what is often referred to as a built-in institutional bias, but a 1999 Supreme Court ruling called the Olmstead Decision is causing a major shake-up. This ruling states that if a person is Medicaid-eligible, which means they meet very strict income guidelines, they must be given the opportunity to have care provided in the least restrictive environment possible, and that more often than not is the home and surrounding community. States and localities are scrambling to have more home and community-based services available to meet the anticipated demand. In large part, we have the very vocal disability community to thank for this significant change.

I took care of my 91-year-old mother and my disabled sister. Think how much money my 6½ years of caregiving saved the system in nursing home fees.

Judy Sing, MaComb, OH

Nursing home care costs on average $50,000 a year, sometimes twice as much in major metropolitan areas. Since Medicaid was specifically designed for low-income individuals and families who do not have insurance or resources to pay for their healthcare, middle-income people have truly been caught in the middle: Medicare provides no long-term care services at all and Medicaid only provides it for a strictly defined population. To make the situation more equitable for the middle class, Congress established rules for long-term care that allow individuals to "spend down" their assets and thereby qualify for assistance. It used to be that when a two-person household was involved, as when a husband and wife are both alive, this practice left the well spouse (often referred to as the community spouse) in poverty, without enough income or assets to cover even her own basic needs. Now, because of changes in the law that came about from the efforts of advocates for the elderly, community spouses are allowed to maintain $2,175 a month of income, $87,000 in assets, and their house and car and still be eligible for payment of nursing home fees according to January 2001 guidelines. This doesn't exactly solve the problem of long-term care financing but it is an improvement.

Workplace-based Health Insurance

Most of us who are eligible for neither Medicare nor Medicaid get our health insurance through our employers. Large employers, because of their strong buying power, can usually negotiate significant savings and more benefits for their employees than smaller ones. Some employers cover the full cost of health insurance for their employees but that number is declining. Others pay a partial amount and, as healthcare premiums go up as they are doing now, employees are being asked to pay more and more of the premiums out of their own pocket. Self-employed individuals often have to find creative ways to obtain reasonably priced health insurance. Some people, such as those who work part-time (many moms of children with special needs fit into this category) may not have the option of employee-offered benefits, and therefore must find a way to pay for individual policies or go without coverage at all.

Caregiving families who received their health insurance through their loved one's employer know the devastating impact that the loss of health insurance can bring. The entire family is left up the proverbial creek having to fend for itself in the rising-cost waters of non-employer-based policies. Even if the caregiver can subsequently obtain coverage from her employer, her loved one, because of his now pre-existing condition, may be caught without any insurance at all. Caregivers themselves who stop working in order to meet their caregiving responsibilities are in the exact same boat when it comes to finding a new, affordable policy.

In the summer of 2001, while preparing to give testimony before the Senate Subcommittee on Oversight of Government Management Restructuring and the District of Columbia regarding the health insurance issues facing the caregiving community, I sent a query to a random selection of caregivers on the NFCA e-mail list, asking them to share their thoughts and experiences regarding health insurance. Some people were just thrilled that I even brought up the subject, since it is so seldom talked about. Others sent in very poignant accounts of what has happened to them and their families and I included a number of them in my testimony. The following comments are typical:

I quit work to care for my husband and paid an exorbitant amount for COBRA insurance for both of us. When that ran out, I had to get an individual policy (which he was not eligible for) and pay for it myself.

Janet Miesiak, Allen Park, MI

I have been caregiver for my mother and aunt, both in their 80s, since 1991. I had to quit my job last year when my mother had another heart attack. I lost health, dental, vision, and disability insurance, plus pension and deferred compensation. I am presently retaining my health insurance through COBRA, but it costs me $304 per month and it will run out . . .

Sandra Jacobson, Bellevue, WA

It's Not Just an Issue of Healthcare Coverage

It would be bad enough if healthcare coverage were the only issue that family caregivers had to deal with, but unfortunately it isn't. There are many other consequences of being a family caregiver in America today. None of us as individuals can address them alone but, by speaking with a united voice, we can bring our concerns to the attention of local communities, states, and the federal government. Then caregiving families will have a chance at a quality of life that is comparable to that of the non-caregiving majority of Americans.

Family Caregivers are Literally Underpinning our Healthcare System

I think the economic benefit that family caregivers provide is underestimated. Before I took over care of my parents, they were in the doctor's office at least once a week.

Wendy Wharton, Oak View, CA

Family caregivers provide over eighty percent of all home care services. The market value of the services provided by family caregivers was estimated to be 257 billion dollars a year in 2002. Family caregivers are literally underpinning our healthcare system and are an irreplaceable resource. Virtually all of the country's functionally disabled seniors receive some of their care from family caregivers, and almost two thirds receive all of their care from family or friends. As you would expect, children with special needs predominately get their care from one or both parents.

Family Caregivers Put Their Own Health at Risk, Sometimes in Dramatic Ways

Family caregivers are known to have a much higher incidence of depression than the rest of the population, and some studies have shown that depression among family caregivers is deeper and lasts longer than the depression experienced by others. Family caregivers often suffer from significant sleep disorders and back problems. Medical studies have shown that the stress of caregiving can cause caregivers' immune systems to function more slowly and thereby increase wound healing time. Other medical studies have shown that elderly caregivers under extreme stress have almost a two-thirds higher mortality rate than non-caregivers and caregivers who don't experience significant stress. Family caregivers, of course, don't need statistics to tell them about the physical and emotional impacts of caregiving. They have their own experiences.

> *Stephanie was born with one quarter of one kidney. Although most new moms don't get a lot of sleep, I virtually got none because of her interventions and reactions to medication. After three months I had lost twenty pounds, had terrible bags under my eyes, and looked like a zombie. The doctor threatened to hospitalize me because I was suffering from exhaustion. When I started thinking it would be a nice break I knew I was in trouble.*
>
> Lauren Agoratus, Mercerville, NJ

My husband recently died from chronic pulmonary disease. He was only 52. I am 43. Shortly after his death I was rushed to the hospital suffering from a severe lack of potassium. I nearly died. I had been so busy caring for Michael and continuing to work, I didn't realize how much I had neglected my own health. I didn't realize what a drain caregiving had been.

Hope C., Prescott, AZ

It's Expensive to Be a Caregiving Family

I spend $600–800 on home care aide services every month and that's because I was able to find a non-certified aide who works for me directly. It would cost me more than twice as much if I went through an agency.

Evie Rosen, Edwards, CO

Families in which one member has a disability spend two and one-half times more on out-of-pocket medical expenses than do non-caregiving families, over eleven percent of their income. This is not surprising when you consider the cost of products and services such as diapers for school-age children and incontinent adults, construction of ramps, accessible toilets, first-floor bedrooms or mother-in-law suites, respite care, and personal attendant aides.

[My wish] is to have the legislature mandate that health insurance companies cover the expense of incontinence supplies. In our case, the yearly cost is $1,500–$1,800.

Sheue Yann Cheng, Potomac, MD

Covering these costs is even harder when a family's income has been reduced because either the caregiver or care receiver has become a part-time employee, turned down a promotion, or left the workforce entirely. When that happens not only is income reduced, but so are potential future pension benefits and social security payments. Caregivers are very often put in an untenable financial position and may not even realize the full impact of it until they themselves need care. Financial concerns are worrisome for most caregiving families, but seem to be worst for parents of children with special needs, many of whom are now living on into adulthood and even old age. Who is going to be able to support these children when their parents are no longer alive?

Caregiving Beyond the Family

Caregivers at Work

Not only are the repercussions of caregiving affecting families in their personal lives, they are also having a profound effect on them in the workplace. Companies both large and small are trying to find ways to keep productivity up while simultaneously giving employees the flexibility they need to care for their ill or disabled loved ones.

The majority of family caregivers are employed outside the home. The NAC/AARP study referred to earlier found that almost two-thirds of America's family caregivers are employed, with fifty-two percent working full time. Businesses are very concerned about the growing number of people involved in caregiving, and rightly so. They are losing billions of dollars a year, as much as twenty-nine billion, because of it. Some of the cost is due to increased absenteeism, reduced productivity on the job, and the costs associated with replacing workers who quit.

Approximately six percent of U.S. businesses have workplace programs to help family caregivers meet their familial responsibilities and still be productive workers. Ironically though, many caregivers at these companies don't take advantage of the programs that are available to them. Some just don't believe that you should bring your personal life to work; others are concerned that by telling their manager about their personal situation they may place their job in jeopardy. There is some evidence to support this concern. In her column on work and family issues for the *Wall Street Journal* of September 13, 2000, Sue Shellenbarger wrote:

> Many readers who responded to a recent column on workplace discrimination against caregivers to the elderly and disabled had their own stories of being treated badly at work because of caregiving duties.
>
> Among about 50 readers who responded, several said they had to lie to gain the flexibility they needed. Others were forced to quit their jobs.

There is no question that our personal lives affect our work lives. We can't cut ourselves in half and then only take one pant leg out of the closet at a time. For that reason win/win solutions for employees and employers must be found. Unfortunately, I don't think they will be until the highest level of management says family caregivers are valued employees who will be respected and protected from discrimination.

Case in point—Fannie Mae, the country's largest non-bank financial services company (they help make it possible for many people to buy a home), has a very innovative family caregiver support program, and it came about precisely because Fannie Mae's CEO, Frank Raines, got involved. He proposed hiring a geriatric care manager to help employees solve programs related to family caregiving and elder care issues. Mr. Raines realized that Fannie Mae needed to go beyond the flexible scheduling, telecommuting, job sharing, and part-time opportunities that were already in place. Caregivers needed someone who knew the ropes to actually locate resources and help them make decisions.

This corporate commitment to providing employees with real assistance in finding solutions to their caregiving problems is good business. Wouldn't it be nice if more companies followed the Fannie Mae lead? Workplace problems would be one less thing that family caregivers needed to be concerned about.

Caregiving in the Legislative and Public Policy Arena

Caregiving and its consequences are of growing concern to Congress and state legislatures, as well as corporate executives. The first piece of national legislation to recognize the role of families in healthcare was The Family and Medical Leave Act (FMLA), passed in 1993. The FMLA allows an employee, in a fifty-person-plus organization, to take twelve weeks of unpaid leave from work because of their own health needs or the health needs of a family member and still retain their job. Research by the National Partnership, the organization behind the FMLA, has shown that the main reason people who would like to take advantage of the program don't is that they just can't afford to give up their paycheck during the time they'd be taking care of things at home. The National Partnership is actively working to find ways for employees to be compensated during their time off and to expand the benefits to employees at smaller companies.

As noted earlier, in 1999 the Supreme Court issued a ruling that has significant meaning for caregiving families. The ruling says that individuals who are eligible for Medicaid must be allowed to get their care at home and in the community if that is what they want. The impact of this ruling is that states and local communities have to beef up the availability of services and resources to meet the needs of the disabled community from infancy through old age. A preliminary report was issued in December 2001 that outlined the Bush administration's proposals for 2002 in response to the Olmstead decision. A section specifically on caregiver support includes plans to enhance and expand respite services.

Too impatient to wait for Congress, Oregon, Wisconsin, and Nebraska have implemented legislation establishing statewide lifespan respite programs. In these states, lifespan respite provides a coordinated system of accessible community-based respite care services for caregivers regardless of age, race, ethnicity, special need, or situation. Other states, such as Oklahoma, have implemented similar programs without legislation, while still others, such as Maryland, have put in place the mechanisms needed for building local systems to assist caregivers in gaining access to lifespan respite programs. While all of this state-based activity has been going on, the National Respite Coalition has been at work trying to gain passage of a national lifespan respite bill introduced in the spring of 2002.

Also more than twenty-five years ago at the state level, California established the Family Caregiver Alliance (FCA) to conduct research, provide and disseminate information, and work to improve the lives of family caregivers of brain-injured adults. California also funds a system of caregiver resource centers throughout the state to help family caregivers on a more local level. In addition, the state gives a $500 tax credit to qualifying caregivers.

Other states provide innovative caregiver support programs too, although not as extensively as California. But, as with all state-funded programs, they can only serve a small percentage of the population needing their help. New Jersey, Pennsylvania, and New York have all been cited as having innovative programs.

Two thousand was a very exciting year for family caregivers. That's when Congress passed, and President Clinton signed into law, the National Family Caregivers Support Program (NFCSP). This was the very first piece of national legislation that specifically provided support services for family caregivers. It called for the establishment of programs, administered through Area Agencies on Aging, to educate, support, train, and provide respite to family caregivers.

Legislation to make Medicare more responsive to the needs of the chronically ill and calling for caregiver education has been introduced into Congress, as have bills to direct Medicare to take caregiver safety and well-being into account when deciding on equipment reimbursement. In recognition that caregiving families have expenses over and above those of non-caregiving families, a $3,000 tax credit for caregiving families has also been proposed. Most recently, legislation to create a lifespan respite program was introduced to make it easier for family caregivers to get the breaks from caregiving that they so greatly need.

These and other actions on the state and national level all point to a growing awareness of the needs of family caregivers and the realization that, although caregiving is an issue families deal with on a very personal level, society needs to support family caregivers and address the consequences of their role on a community and governmental level. For the promise of past initiatives to turn into expanded and ongoing programs in the future, family caregivers need to become involved in the debate and speak up for what they and their loved ones need. In a representative democracy such as ours, the stories and voices of constituents make a difference and influence the outcome of legislation.

What Do We Do?

Do you believe the negative consequences of caregiving are fair? Do you believe that love and responsibility should be penalized rather than rewarded? I don't.

Do you think that more businesses need to be caregiver friendly and that other caregiver-friendly legislation should be enacted at the state and federal level? I definitely do.

I think caregiving families should have access to a care coordinator who can help them bridge the gap between the fear they experience and the adaptation that they face when crises hit, regardless of the age of their care recipient. I think Medicare needs to be overhauled to reflect the reality of our lives and the needs of the chronically ill as well as those with acute conditions. I also think that caregivers should have input into the design of community-based programs aimed at helping them and their loved ones, and that medical education needs to be reformed so that doctors have a greater understanding of how to work constructively with family caregivers. I think many things need to be done to create a more level playing field for caregiving families as they confront the game of life.

I know of course that life isn't fair. We are all dealt a hand at birth and events intercede in both wonderful and horrific ways. I also know that the negative consequences of caregiving were never intended and have come about because of a confluence of discoveries and circumstances. All the more reason that we should strive to reduce the impact of caregiving on individuals, families, and society. In fact, now that we are aware of the inequities I believe we ought to try to correct them, not only for our own sakes, but also for all of the caregivers who will follow us.

I suspect many of you are saying "I don't even have time to take a relaxing bath in peace. How do you expect me to get involved in changing the world?" I don't. I'm only asking that you start to think about helping to make life better for your loved one and yourself. That's really not any different than what I've been suggesting throughout this entire book. I'm just asking you to think about it in a slightly different way now.

I'm suggesting that you acknowledge your role as a family caregiver. What I mean by that statement is this: It is important to recognize that although our love and sense of responsibility, our belief in the Ten Commandments, our marriage vows, and the very fact that we are parents are what compel us to care for our chronically ill, disabled, or aged family member, partner, or good friend, the job of family caregiving often demands an excessively high price that far exceeds what a just and compassionate society should ask of its citizens.

Moving from the concept that caregiving is strictly a personal issue not to be talked about in public to the belief that all caregivers are part of a very large and ever-growing constituency that deserves recognition by others does not require time or energy-draining action. It does however require thought and consideration of the information laid out in this book. If you can do just that, if you can acknowledge to yourself that you are a family caregiver, you will already be making a difference. Research has shown that family caregivers who self-identify as caregivers are known to be more proactive in support of their loved one, more confident in talking with their loved one's doctor, more apt to be concerned about their own welfare, somewhat less isolated, and definitely more cognizant of the connection between their personal caregiving and its broader social issues. The very act of self-identifying can begin to increase your ability to be an effective, healthy caregiver and a concerned citizen.

If you do have some time and energy to spare, if you are sufficiently upset about the current state of affairs that caregiving families find themselves in, you can move beyond acknowledgement to action.

- You can try to read more articles or listen with more attention to the TV news when healthcare issues are being discussed. Just by being better informed you are making a difference.
- You can discuss what you've read or heard with others and thereby hear someone else's point of view. And they can begin to consider yours.
- If you are part of a support group, you can suggest that the

group talk about a specific topic of concern and write a letter to your state or federal representative.

- You can ask your faith community to say prayers not only for those who are ill, but also for their family caregivers and you can suggest that the congregation consider establishing care teams to help out caregiving families during times of crisis.
- You can find out if the voluntary health agency that is focused on your loved one's condition is actively working on issues that are important to you and offer to be part of a letter writing or telephone campaign.
- You can agree to share your story with the media so that the general public can gain a clearer picture of what caregivers' lives are really like.
- You can try to join a local community coalition advising your county on caregiver-related issues.
- You can become part of a caregiver support organization and expand your knowledge, lessen your loneliness, and assist them in their efforts to provide information and support and to bring about social and legislative changes to help you and your loved one.
- You can do one or more of these things depending upon your time and your inclination. Each one will make a difference.

But first you have to accept that family caregiving goes beyond you and me. You have to be willing to stand up and be counted as one of the whole, one family caregiver among millions, who is not alone, who wants to take charge of life, who is comfortable with the concept of self-care, and who values and honors the caregiving work being done. You need to be the type of family caregiver who can recognize your own strengths, but can also admit you need help, and be willing to ask for it and accept it when it is offered.

If we all just do that, so much is possible.

Afterword

It's been almost thirty years since Steven was diagnosed with multiple sclerosis, and more than a dozen years since Cindy and I began to talk about finding a way to help family caregivers. I never could have imagined at either of those times how each event would affect my life and those of so many other people.

I am grateful for how I have grown as a person because of both of these events, and I am humbled by the achievements of NFCA and the knowledge that the organization Cindy and I began has become a national force for education, support, empowerment, and advocacy for America's family caregivers.

I look back at what has occurred, both the good and the bad, and I look forward to the future with hope and an eye on reality.

Cindy's mom Madeleine died in 1996, so Cindy is now a member of the "post-caregiver" contingent. Her grieving experiences during the first year after Madeleine's death gave us first-hand knowledge upon which to draw when we created a series of five bereavement articles for former caregivers.

Cindy and her husband Rich moved to California in the summer of 2001 to be closer to their daughter, son-in-law, and especially their grandson, but she remains on the NFCA board and continues to use her wonderful graphic talent to help communicate NFCA's message. Although we can't do it in person anymore, we continue to have a weekly lunch date. Now it is by phone, and for Cindy it is actually breakfast, not lunch, but no matter. We continue to collaborate and coordinate and build our friendship and the good work of NFCA with the help of so many others, and the generous support of individuals, foundations, and corporations.

Steven, of course, does not get better. That is the way of MS. There is always the slow, slithering deterioration of his abilities. But I know we are lucky, that his condition could have progressed much faster than it has, and I am optimistic about our future. When we bought our current house, I didn't think we would be able to stay in it as long as we have, and now we are projecting that it will meet our needs, no matter how much Steven's disability progresses, for as long we feel comfortable staying in it. Steven is looking toward retirement in a couple of years, unless the MS insists it be sooner. That will be a big change, and I know we will integrate it into our lives as we have others, with some bumps along the way.

Life is about change, the ones we initiate and others that come roaring into our lives like an avalanche, unplanned and unwanted. How we deal with all of them is what matters. And so I will continue to go forth, hopefully taking the lessons I have learned to heart and using them to make a better day for Steven and myself, and for the millions of other people who are family caregivers today and the millions more that will follow them.

A Short List of Helpful Contacts

The National Family Caregivers Association (NFCA) receives hundreds of phone calls and e-mails a week from family caregivers seeking resources, referrals, and advice. The following list includes much of the same information we provide to caregivers over the phone.

A Good Place to Start

It's always wise to find out what your county and state have to offer in the way of services, even if you think you won't qualify for them. Check the blue pages of your phone book for the numbers, or go on-line. Counties and states all have Web sites. Type the name of your state, or county and state, into any major search engine (e.g. Iowa, or Montgomery County, Pennsylvania). Navigate from there to locate the Department of Health and Human Services and the specific office most relevant to your needs, such as the office on disabilities, elder affairs, or maternal and child health.

Other good sources of information include your local hospital or clinic (social work department), area adult day centers, social service and faith-based agencies, and/or the local chapter of the health agency that focuses on your loved one's condition. It is by no means certain that any of these will offer caregiver support services, but they are good places to check, and they are good sources for information about services that may directly support your loved one.

Caregiver Organizations, Information, Advocacy, and Support Resources

Children of Aging Parents (CAPS)
1609 Woodbourne Road #302A
Levittown, PA 19057
800-227-7294
Web: www.careguide.net

CAPS assists caregivers of the elderly with information and referrals, a network of support groups, and publications and programs that promote public awareness of the value and the needs of family caregivers.

Family Caregiver Alliance (FCA)
690 Market Street
Suite 600
San Francisco, CA 94104
415-434-3388
800-445-8106 (CA only)
Web: www.caregiver.org
e-mail: info@caregiver.org

FCA is the lead agency in California's system of Caregiver Resource Centers. FCA provides support and help to family caregivers, and champions their cause through education, services, research, and advocacy. Services are specific to CA. Information can be accessed nationally.

Family Voices
PO Box 769
Algodones, NM 87001
888-835-5669
Web: www.familyvoices.org
e-mail: kidshealth@familyvoices.org

Offers information on healthcare policies relevant to children
with special needs in every state.

Friends Health Connection
PO Box 114
New Brunswick, NJ 08903
800-483-7436
Web: www.48friend.org
e-mail: FHC@pilot.NJIN.NET

Links persons with illness or disability and their family caregivers with others experiencing the same challenges.

National Alliance for Caregiving
4720 Montgomery Lane, Suite 642
Bethesda, MD 20814
301-718-8444
Web: www.caregiving.org

Although not an organization directly for caregivers, NAC's
Web site helps family caregivers learn about Web sites, videos,
pamphlets, etc., that have been reviewed and approved as providing solid information.

National Family Caregivers Association
10400 Connecticut Avenue, Suite 500
Kensington, MD 20895
800-896-3650
Web: www.nfcacares.org
e-mail: info@nfcacares.org

The National Family Caregivers Association (NFCA) is a grassroots organization designed to educate, support, empower, and speak up for the millions of Americans who care for chronically ill, aged, or disabled loved ones. NFCA is the only constituency organization that reaches across the boundaries of different diagnoses, different relationships, and different life stages to address the common needs and concerns of all family caregivers. NFCA serves as a public voice for family caregivers to the press, to Congress, and to the general public. NFCA offers publications, information, referral services, caregiver support, and advocacy.

Rosalynn Carter Institute (RCI)
Georgia Southwestern University
800 Wheatley Street
Americus, GA 31709
912-928-1234
Web: www.rci.gsw.edu

RCI provides educational programs for family and professional caregivers, conducts research, and disseminates caregiving information.

Well Spouse Foundation
PO Box 30093
Elkins Park, PA 19027
800-838-0879
Web: www.wellspouse.org
e-mail: info@wellspouse.org

A national membership organization that gives support to husbands, wives, and partners of the chronically ill and/or disabled, Well Spouse has a network of support groups and also a newsletter for spouses.

Caregiver Web Sites

There are a variety of Web sites that offer information and support for family caregivers in addition to those from specific organizations. Because Web sites come and go, especially commercial ones, we are listing here only those that have been around for a substantial period of time and that we are fairly sure will continue to be live for the foreseeable future. To find other sites just type caregiver, caregivers, or family caregiving into a search engine. Many site addresses will be displayed.

www.caregiver.com
www.caregiver911.org
www.caregiving.com

Caring for Elders

General Recommendations

Contact your county office of senior services or elder affairs, area adult day centers, and/or social service agencies providing services to the elderly. Check blue pages of your phone book or type the name of your county and state into an Internet search engine.

Referral and Information Sources

AARP
601 E Street, NW
Washington, DC 20049
800-424-3410
Web: www.aarp.org

Supplies education and information about caregiving, long-term care, and aging, including publications and audio-visual aids for caregivers.

Christopher and Dana Reeve Paralysis Resource Center
636 Morris Turnpike
Short Hills, NJ 07078
800-539-7309
Web: www.paralysis.org

The Center provides a comprehensive trustworthy source of information for people living with paralysis and their caregivers to promote health, foster involvement in the community, and improve quality of life.

Eldercare Locator
National Association of Area Agencies on Aging
927 Fifteenth Street, NW 6th Floor
Washington, DC 20005
800-677-1116
Web: www.n4a.org.

Provides referrals to Area Agencies on Aging via zip code locations. Offers information about many eldercare issues and services in local communities.

The National Association of Professional Geriatric Care Managers
1604 North Country Club Road
Tucson, AZ 85716
520-881-800-8
Web: www.caremanager.org

Geriatric care managers (GCMs) are health care professionals, most often social workers, who help families in dealing with the problems and challenges associated with caring for the elderly. This national organization will refer you to their state chapters, which in turn can give you the names of GCMs in your area. This information is also available on-line.

U.S. Administration on Aging
330 Independence Avenue, SW
Washington, DC 20201
202-619-7501
Web: www.aoa.gov

This government Web site has a special section on family caregiving.

End of Life Planning, Hospice, and Bereavement Information

Aging with Dignity
PO Box 1661
Tallahassee, FL 32302-1661
888 -594 7437
Web: www.agingwithdignity.org

Aging with Dignity publishes the Five Wishes Living Will document, a very user friendly and comprehensive document that is legal in at least thirty-three states and the District of Columbia.

Last Acts
Web: www.lastacts.org

Last Acts is a major public education initiative of the Robert Wood Johnson Foundation focused on improving end of life care for Americans by impacting medical and public education and more. The Web site is very comprehensive.

National Hospice Foundation
2001 S Street NW
Washington, DC 20009
800-854-3402
Web: www.hospicefoundation.org

Hosts an annual teleconference on issues of bereavement, and has publications on grief and bereavement.

National Hospice and Palliative Care Organization
1700 Diagonal Road
Alexandria, VA 22314
800-658-8898
Web: www.nhpco.org

Operates a hospice help line to provide the general public and healthcare providers with information.

The Compassionate Friends
PO Box 3696
Oakbrook, IL 60522
877-969-0010
Web: www.compassionatefriends.org

Offers telephone support and understanding to families that have lost a child. Maintains a resource library and has a national chapter network and newsletter.

Health Insurance, Prescription Drug, and Medical Care Support and Information Programs

General Recommendations

Contact your county or state Department of Health and Human Services, or area social service agencies, such as Catholic Charities, Association of Jewish Family and Children's Agencies, and local chapters of voluntary health agencies to find out if they offer any financial support programs and how to apply for them. Unfortunately, there are not nearly as many programs as there are people who need them.

Federal Hill-Burton Free Care Program
800-638-0742 (message center)

Provides referrals to agencies that offer free medical care.

HealthInsurance.com
3030 South Bundy Drive
Los Angeles, CA 90066
310-737-9300
Web: www.healthinsurance.com

Fairly new Web site that provides consumers and small businesses with quotes for health insurance. May help those who have lost their health insurance find an affordable alternative.

Medicare Rights Center
1460 Broadway, 11th Floor
New York, NY 10036
212-869-3859
888-HMO-9050
Web: www.medicarerights.org

Provides hotlines for direct services, education/training, policy, and media relations for both Medicare and Medicaid.

Medicine Program
PO Box 520
Doniphan, MO 63935
573-996-7300
Web: www.themedicineprogram.com

A means-tested program for persons who do not have coverage either through insurance or government subsidies for outpatient prescription drugs, and who cannot afford to purchase medications at retail prices.

National Patient Advocates Foundation
753 Thimble Shoals, Suite B
Newport News, VA 23606
800-532-5274
Web: www.patientadvocate.org

The Patient Advocates Foundation serves as a liaison between patients and their insurers, employers, and/or creditors to resolve insurance, job discrimination, and/or debt crisis matters relating to patient's condition.

Organizations for Those with Rare Disorders

Referral Sources

National Information Center
Orphan Drugs & Rare Diseases
PO Box 1133
Washington, DC 20013-1133
800-336-4749

Provides an information hotline and nationwide referral service to additional resources, including support groups.

National Organization for Rare Disorders
100 Route 37
PO Box 8923
New Fairfield, CT 06812
800-999-6673
Web: www.rarediseases.org

Serves as an information clearinghouse on rare diseases and orphan drugs; provides referrals to resources that offer support and assistance to people with rare disorders and to their families.

Home Care Agencies, Assisted Living, and Nursing Homes

Watchdog Agencies

Consumer Consortium on Assisted Living
PO Box 3375
Arlington, VA 22203
703-841-2333
Web: www.ccal.org

CCAL is a national consumer-focused organization that is dedicated to representing the needs of residents in assisted living facilities and educating consumers, professionals, and the general public about assisted living issues. Their book "Choosing an Assisted Living Facility, Strategies for Making the Right Decision" provides helpful information and contains a concise questionnaire.

National Citizens Coalition for Nursing Home Reform
1424 Sixteenth Street, NW, Suite 202
Washington, DC 20036
202-332-2275
Web: www.nccnhr.org
e-mail: nccnhr@nccnhr.org

Serves as an information clearinghouse; offers referrals nation-wide for help with concerns about long-term care facilities.

Referral Sources

National Association for Home Care
228 Seventh Street, SE
Washington, DC 20003
202-547-7424
Web: www.nahc.org

Organization for home healthcare agency providers, but also includes Internet links for consumers to access a list of their member agencies across the country.

New Lifestyles
800-869-9549
Web: www.NewLifeStyles.com

Publishes regional directories of nursing homes, assisted living, and retirement communities. Call for a free copy or visit them on the Web.

Senior Alternatives
800-350-0770
Web: www.senioralternatives.com

Publishes regional directories of nursing homes, assisted living, and retirement communities. Call for a free copy or visit them on the Web.

Visiting Nurses Association of America
11 Beacon Street, Suite 910
Boston, MA 02108
617-523-4042
Web: www.vnaa.org
e-mail: vnaa@vnaa.org

Promotes community based home healthcare. You can contact them to find your local VNA.

Medical Transport and Hospitality Housing

Referral Resources

National Association of Hospital Hospitality Houses
(NAHHH)
PO Box 18087
Ashville, NC 28814-0087
800-542-9730
Web: www.nahhh.org

Represents organizations that provide lodging (and service) for families receiving medical care away from home; furnishes information about hospitality homes in caller's area; offers newsletter; publishes annual directory of facilities offering lodging.

National Patient Air Transport Helpline
Mercy Medical Airlift
4620 Haygood Road, Suite 1
Virginia Beach, VA 23455
800-296-1217
Web: www.PatientTravel.org

Offers help in locating air transportation for needy patients who need distant specialized medical evaluation, diagnosis, or treatment. NPATH is the central consumer referral source for all major medical transport providers.

Respite Resources

National Organizations, Programs, and Referral Sources

Easter Seals
230 West Monroe Street, Suite 1800
Chicago, IL 60606
800-221-6827
Web: www.easter-seals.org
e-mail: info@easter-seals.org

Provides a variety of services at 400 sites nationwide for children and adults with disabilities, including adult day care, in-home care, camps for children with special needs and more. Services vary by site.

Family Friends
National Council on the Aging, Inc.
409 Third Street, SW
Washington, DC 20024
202-479-6675 or 202-479-6672
Web: www.ncoa.org

Provides respite (and other services) for families of children with special needs by men and women volunteers over the age of 50. Programs located throughout the country—with 47 centers and over 2000 volunteers.

National Association of Adult Day Services
8201 Greensboro Drive
Suite 300

McLean, VA 22102
1-866-890-7357
Web: www.nadsa.org

Provides information about locating adult day care centers in your local area.

National Respite Coalition
4016 Oxford Street
Annandale, VA 22003
703-256-9578
Web: www.chtop.com/NRC.htm.
e-mail: jbkagan@nrc.com

NRC provides a list of states that have respite coalitions. These state coalitions then list respite services available in their state. The majority of the information is focused on helping families of children with special needs, but lately there has been an effort to enlarge their referral base to include lifespan respite information. The NRC is working to gain passage of national lifespan respite legislation.

National Respite Locator Service
800 Eastowne Drive, Suite 105
Chapel Hill, NC 27514
800-773-5433
Web: www.chtop.com/locator.htm.

Lists over 1,900 sites nationwide, the vast majority of which focus on respite care for families of children with special needs, but there is an effort to begin to include lifespan information as well.

Shepherd's Centers of America
One West Armour, Suite 201
Kansas City, MO 64111

800-547-7073
Web: www.shepherdcenters.org
e-mail: staff@shepherdcenters.org

Provides respite care, telephone visitors, in-home visitors, nursing home visitors, home health aides, support groups, adult day care, and information and referrals for accessing other services available in the community. Services vary by center. There are currently seventy-five centers around the country.

Voluntary Health Agencies

This list is provided by the National Health Council.

Alzheimer's Association
800-272-3900
Web: www.alz.org

American Autoimmune Related Diseases Association
800-598-4668
Web: www.aarda.org

American Cancer Society
800-ACS-2345
Web: www.cancer.org

American Diabetes Association
800-342-2383
Web: www.diabetes.org

American Foundation for AIDS Research (amfAR)
800-392-6327
Web: www.amfar.org

American Heart Association, National Center
800-AHA-USA1 (242-8721)
Web: www.americanheart.org

American Kidney Fund
Help Line: 800-638-8299
Web: www.kidneyfund.org

American Liver Foundation
800-GO-LIVER (465-4837)
(888) 4-HEP-ABC (443-7222)
Web: www.liverfoundation.org

American Lung Association®
Toll-free number to connect to local
American Lung Association offices: 800-LUNG-USA
Web: www.lungusa.org

American Tinnitus Association
800-634-8978
Web: www.ata.org

Amyotrophic Lateral Sclerosis Association
800-782-4747
Web: www.alsa.org

Arthritis Foundation
800-283-7800
Web: www.arthritis.org

Asthma & Allergy Foundation of America
800-7-ASTHMA (727-8462)
Web: www.aafa.org

Cancer Research Foundation of America
800-227-CRFA
Web: www.preventcancer.org
e-mail: sguiffre@CRFA.org

CHADD
(Children and Adults with Attention-Deficit Hyperactivity
Disorder)
800-233-4050
Web: www.chadd.org

Crohn's & Colitis Foundation of America
800-343-3637 (to order brochures and for general information)
Web: www.ccfa.org

Easter Seals
800-221-6827
Web: www.easter-seals.org

Epilepsy Foundation
800-EFA-1000 (800-332-1000)
Web: www.epilepsyfoundation.org

The Foundation Fighting Blindness
888-394-3937
Web: www.blindness.org

Huntington's Disease Society of America
800-345-HDSA
Web: www.hdsa.org

Kidney Cancer Association
800-850-9132
Web: www.kidneycancerassociation.org

The Leukemia & Lymphoma Society
800-955-4572
Web: www.leukemia-lymphoma.org

Lupus Foundation of America
800-558-0121
Web: www.lupus.org

March of Dimes
888-663-4637
Web: www.modimes.org

Myasthenia Gravis Foundation of America
800-541-5454
Web: www.myasthenia.org

Myositis Association of America
800-821-7356
Web: Web: www.myositis.org
e-mail: maa@myositis.org

National Down Syndrome Society
800-221-4602
Web: www.ndss.org

National Hemophilia Foundation
800-42-HANDI (424-2634)
Web: www.hemophilia.org

National Mental Health Association
800-969-NMHA (6642)
Web: www.nmha.org

National Multiple Sclerosis Society
800-FIGHT-MS (344-4867)
Web: www.nationalmssociety.org

National Osteoporosis Foundation
202-223-2226
Web: www.nof.org

National Psoriasis Foundation
800-723-9166
Web: www.psoriasis.org

National Sleep Foundation
202-347-3471
Web: www.sleepfoundation.org

Osteogenesis Imperfecta Foundation
800-981-BONE (2663)
Web: www.oif.org

The Paget Foundation
800-23-PAGET (237-2438)
Web: www.paget.org

Sjogren's Syndrome Foundation
800-4SJOGREN (475-6473)
Web: www.sjogrens.org

Spina Bifida Association of America
800-621-3141
Web: www.sbaa.org

Tourette Syndrome Association, Inc.
888 4-OURET (486-8738)
Web: www.tsa-usa.org

Tuberous Sclerosis Alliance
800-225-6872
Web: www.tsalliance.org

United Ostomy Association
800-826-0826
Web: www.uoa.org

Additional VHAs

American Parkinson Disease Association
800-223-2732
Web: www.apdaparkinson.com

United Cerebral Palsy Associations
1660 L Street, NW
Washington, DC 20036
202-776-0406
Web: www.ucpa.org
e-mail: ucpantl@ucpa.org

Cystic Fibrosis Foundation
6931 Arlington Blvd.
Bethesda, MD 20814
800-344-4823
Web: www.cff.org

Practical Advice and Information from the Professionals: Personal, Medical, Legal, and Financial

Information for these Tip Sheets was researched and compiled by Pat Kaufman and Nancy Carson, contributing writers to *TAKE CARE!*, unless otherwise noted.

PERSONAL CONCERNS: TIP SHEETS ON SUPPORT, SLEEP, AND INTIMACY

Many caregivers want to find a support group. Others want to figure out how they will ever get a good night sleep again, and although not talked about much, many caregivers are concerned about the changes caregiving has wrought on intimacy. The following three tip sheets address these concerns.

― TIP SHEET #1 ―

Looking for a Support Group? Things to Consider

Why a Support Group?

There is broad agreement on what support groups offer. Some benefits are:

- A safe haven for sharing true feelings; a non-judgmental atmosphere.
- A social outlet where you can make new friends.
- Information about reliable products and services.
- A place to learn coping mechanisms, saving you much trial and error.
- Advice on what lies ahead, so you can anticipate changes.
- Support for your sanity and confidence—you are not alone.
- Help in dealing with family members.
- TLC from people who truly understand your situation.

What Makes a Support Group Effective?

While any given group may or may not work for you personally, there are characteristics that make some groups more effective than others. Keep these in mind as you explore your own choices.

- A caring atmosphere and trust between group members.
- A comfortable mix of participants, so bonds can build.
- Clear structure and purpose; members know why we are there and what will happen.
- Agreement on group rules, including confidentiality.
- A good facilitator.

Many groups rely on trained professionals, but the background of the facilitator is less important than his or her ability to devise and use an appropriate structure, identify resources, respect group rules, and offer the empathy and concern that members need.

Types of Support Groups

Support groups can be organized in any number of ways. Although effective support groups have similar characteristics, their organizing structures can be very different. It's important to understand the different forms that support groups can take, so you can decide which best meets your needs.

Condition-Specific Groups

These groups focus on a particular disease, disability, or condition. They may be organized within a hospital structure, or by an organization such as The Spinal Cord Injury Network or the American Stroke Association. They may be open to anyone interested in the condition, or designed for sub-groups, such as patients or family members, or a combination of both. The advantage of disease-specific groups is that they offer access to excellent, up-to-date information on the condition as well as information about local resources.

Caregiver Groups

These groups are founded on the shared experience that comes from being a family caregiver and all the emotions that accompany that role. Because the focus is on the caregiver—not the disease or condition—caregivers can openly discuss their own difficulties. Caregivers seldom take the time or find the place to talk about their own needs, so this type of group may be especially valuable.

Relationship-Oriented Groups

This approach focuses on the relationship of a caregiver to the ill or disabled person as the cornerstone. A group might serve parents of children with special needs, children of aging parents, or spouses of the chronically ill. The special nature of the relationship that each member shares makes for conversations that bring relief and support.

Family-Centered Groups

Closer to a therapy group than a support group, family-centered groups work with the family as a whole, improving communication and striving to strengthen the entire family as it copes with the illness of one of its members. In most cases, these groups require the structure and leadership that comes from having a professional facilitator with special training.

Advocacy Groups

A fairly new trend is for support groups to include some advocacy activities, or to connect with advocacy groups. Following the influence of AIDS activist groups and the response of Congress and other funders to organized campaigns for dollars such as breast cancer research, some support groups have taken on advocacy roles. This can be both a healthy outlet for frustration and energy, and a way to hasten research, educate the media about a particular issue, or influence legislation.

On-line Groups

On-line groups provide many of the same benefits as traditional support groups, but have special characteristics. Worldwide self-help communities are possible, access to information is essentially unlimited, and connections can be made from your home. And for someone in a rural area, or someone dealing with a rare condition, electronic connections may be the only way to be in touch with others sharing your struggle. Relief from isolation has always been a principal benefit of groups. A caregiver who cannot leave home can be a contributing member of an on-line group at any time and in any place.

Questions to Ask

Remember, joining a support group is an experiment. If one group does not work for you, try another, or try the same one

again when the time seems better. Selecting a group that
works in a way that is comfortable for you, and knowing what
to expect, makes a big difference. Here are some questions to
ask:

- Who sponsors/runs the group? A hospital, church, or established organization sponsor is a pretty good indicator
  that there will be an appropriate structure and reliable operation.
- Who is the facilitator? Talk to the leader if possible, and
  outline your concerns and interests. See how the two of
  you relate. Ask about the leader's background and training, and how long the group has been running.
- What is the group's organizing principle? If you are newly
  dealing with a disease or condition, you may need information and resources that a condition-specific group can
  offer. If you have been caregiving for a long time, you may
  need support, shared experiences, and a place to let down
  your hair more than you need information.
- What is the makeup of the group? Where and how often
  does it meet? What is expected of you—is participation
  required, or can you just listen? What are the rules of confidentiality?

How to Find a Group

Support groups do not exist in every community and those
in your area may not meet your needs, but it is always worth
the search. In the process you may make new friends and learn
a great deal about other services in your community.

- The social work department of a hospital is always a good
  place to start. If the hospital itself doesn't run any groups,
  perhaps the person you talk to can suggest where else to
  turn.

- Social service agencies, such as Catholic Charities, Jewish Family and Children's Services, and Lutheran Social Services, often sponsor support groups as part of their community outreach. They tend to be open to all, not just people of a particular faith.
- A voluntary health agency that focuses on your loved one's condition, such as the American Diabetes Association or Epilepsy Foundation, is likely to offer support groups for patients, and they may offer them for family members, as well.
- Your County's Department of Disability and Elder Affairs may offer or know of support groups in your area.
- Caregiver-focused organizations such as Children of Aging Parents or the Well Spouse Foundation, or if you live in California, the Family Caregiver Alliance, are good places to check. You can locate them on the Web by typing the organization's name into any search engine.
- Your church or synagogue may have a series of support groups or be willing to help you start one.

─────────── ⟹ **TIP SHEET #2** ⟸ ───────────

A Good Night's Sleep: The Caregiver's Dream

If you've been feeling moody and unhappy lately, found that you're not as productive as you used to be, or noticed that you're having difficulty concentrating and making decisions, don't be too quick to dismiss these symptoms as the inevitable lot of a harried caregiver. You may be suffering from the very serious effects of sleep deprivation. This can affect your ability to provide care to another and marginalize your own health status.

Facts Worth Noting About Sleep and Sleeplessness

First and foremost is that sleepiness, while it may sound amusing or not serious to some, has been targeted by the National Commission on Sleep Disorders as one of the most significant causes of error and accident throughout our society.

Another little-known fact about sleep is that in the past century Americans have reduced their average nightly total sleep time by about twenty percent, even though there is no evidence that we need less sleep today than our forebears did.

Are You Sleep Deprived? Answer these Questions and Find Out.

Do you get five or fewer hours of sleep per night? Do you consistently short-change your sleep needs?

Studies have shown that restricting sleep to five or fewer hours per night can result in measurable losses in the ability to respond, remember, and react. Even more worrisome is the fact that these problems get worse as your sleep restriction continues day after day. Researchers believe that the vast majority of adults need at least seven hours of sleep per night to avoid the consequences of sleep deprivation.

Have you noticed a decrease in your performance ability? Do you routinely ignore the clock and push yourself beyond your physical resources? Do you figure that if worse comes to worst you can always cut hours out of your sleep time?

Researchers on sleep deprivation have documented actual mental lapses that negatively affect the ability to perform tasks. Other effects of sleepiness include an increase in false responses and a measurable slowing of response time in general, both of which account for a failure to work with normal speed and efficiency.

Are you constantly moody and irritable?

Trying to balance the physical and mental demands of caregiving can make anyone prone to mood swings, so don't judge yourself too harshly. If your degree of moodiness seems out of proportion to your usual ability to cope, your sleep patterns may be a cause.

First Steps Toward Combating the Problem of Sleep Deprivation

- Educate yourself. Just realizing that not getting enough sleep can lead to debilitating consequences will at least make you more open to finding ways to improve your sleep patterns.
- Realize that medical professionals are rarely trained to identify sleep problems. Often there's no one to turn to because the medical profession has been slow to recognize sleep disorders. Knowing that your doctor may not be tuned in to sleep disorders, you may want to take the initiative by bringing up the problem and asking for a referral to a more knowledgeable source.
- Try to identify the source of your problem and make changes.
- If the problems stem from your loved one's physical condition, is there anything that can be done so that he or she doesn't have to rely on you so much during the night? If the problem is the need to go to the bathroom, might a bedside commode, a catheter, or even a diaper solve the problem, at least sometimes? If you can't think of a way to solve the problem, try discussing it with another caregiver. Sometimes the experience of others provides the best advice.

Alternative Solutions

If you've tried to eliminate or ameliorate the cause of the problem and nothing helps, look at what changes you can make in your own behavioral patterns. If your resources allow, consider hiring a home care aide to sleep over once or twice during the week, or even for just a couple of hours in the afternoon so that you can take a nap.

If money is tight and you cannot afford outside help, this may be the time to call a family meeting and ask for help from others. No family in the area? Consider this: If you are a member of a church or synagogue, talk to your priest or rabbi. Find out if members of the congregation might be willing to pitch in from time to time to help you get a complete night's sleep. Or consider this: Is it possible to get your care recipient out of the house during the day, to an adult day care center, or even for a drive with a neighbor, just to give you time for a cat nap?

None of these suggestions may be the right solution for you, but the point to recognize is that you may need to be creative in finding a way to help yourself. Lack of sleep is a true health hazard. Getting adequate sleep is a necessity, not a luxury, especially for family caregivers.

TIP SHEET #3

Intimacy: A Casualty of Caregiving

There is a hidden cost to caregiving. It's not a financial expense, although you may be paying a pretty steep price. It's measured in emotional currency and there are no insurance policies to guarantee you protection. What is it? It's the price you pay when illness or disability disrupts your normal family patterns and deprives you of the comfortable intimacy you previously enjoyed.

What is Intimacy?

Between spouses, it has a sexual dimension. Among all family members, intimacy becomes tangible in the caring and understanding acts that reassure family members that a safe and loving place exists for them.

How Caregiving Affects Intimacy? Things to Think About

While everyone is different, caregivers do share some common experiences in the way their intimate relationships are affected. Depending on which member of the family is ill or disabled, intimacy can suffer in a number of ways.

Altered Roles, Altered Images

It's hard to think of your dad as a tower of strength when he has been weakened by heart disease. It's hard to think of your spouse as a lover when you have to help her eat. If you were the primary breadwinner and all of a sudden you are expected to become the primary bread-maker, that's not only a role change. It requires a shift in consciousness.

Loss of Sexual Intimacy

It's hard enough to talk about sexual problems in the best of times; when illness or disability is added to the equation it sometimes seems impossible. Loss of sexual intimacy because a spouse is ill or disabled is a big issue, and it is the one we think of first when the question of sex and disability arises. However, sexual intimacy gets lost in many other caregiving situations, as well.

When a parent moves in with you and your family it is not unusual to be self-conscious about sex. It can almost be as if you are a kid again looking over your shoulder to make sure your parents haven't come home early.

When a child is born with a significant disability or becomes ill, sex may well be the last thing anyone can think of after endless days of endless tasks. Mates can quickly lose their appeal under the strain of being members of a special needs family.

Loss of Balance

Most families have their own internal mechanisms that keep life predictable and promote harmony and intimacy.

Caregiving, with its added demands on time and energy, can shatter that equilibrium. The tension it produces is not conducive to quiet time and intimate conversations.

How to Re-establish Intimacy

Sailing in such uncharted emotional waters, it's difficult to know how to respond to the new, often overwhelming situations that confront you as a caregiver. Everyone's personality and coping mechanisms are unique, and the challenges of caregiving can bring out the worst and the best in a caregiver, sometimes all in the space of a few hours. Still, there are ways to bring balance back to your life and break the negative patterns that sap the intimacy from caregiving families. Looking again at the common problems, here are some suggestions for dealing with them.

Accept the New Realities

Intimacy can't survive shrouded in anger or denial. In order to reestablish bonds or build new ones, you and others, including the care recipient, must come to terms with the cards life has dealt.

Enhance Independence

Beware of over-protectiveness. It's important to encourage your care recipient to carry as many roles as possible, to develop a new sense of self-esteem when one has been lost. You can't return things to normal, or make your life like that of non-caregiving families, but you can look for ways that allow you to have a relationship that isn't based solely on one person giving and the other receiving.

Share Enjoyable Activities

Intimacy comes from shared experiences, private jokes, and special occasions. You may be able to find new ways to enjoy old activities, albeit differently than before. You can try to find new activities to share that don't require lost abilities. You can create special times that carry a meaning only for you and your care recipient or other close friends or family members. It's not what you do. It's the fact that you do something.

Regaining Sexual Intimacy

No one needs to tell you that caregivers and their intimate partners are generally reluctant to discuss problems with sexual relations. In some cases, such as when a caregiver is concerned about catching something from the loved one, the problems can go away with a little education. At other times, some creative scheduling can help a child of an aging parent or parents of a child with special needs create a window of privacy in which uninhibited intimacy can flourish. When the problem is more basic and one partner is no longer capable of sexual activity, the solutions are never simple.

Develop a Larger View of Intimacy

Sex is only a part of it. Ordinary expressions of affection, such as kissing and hugging, still remain important and desirable, even if new modes of doing so have to be found. The first step is getting the problem out on the table. If it is hard for you to say what you are thinking and feeling outright, try writing it down and handing your loved one a note. For some people talking to a therapist can help, with or without their partner present. This is territory that is complicated and personal. There are no right answers; there are simply answers that are right for you.

Regaining balance

Although caregiving can be pervasive, you don't want it to be all-consuming, allowing your energies to become so depleted that you're too tired or too resentful to even try to restore family intimacy. Intimacy doesn't just happen. It requires an effort, and therefore you have to decide how important it is to you to have an intimate relationship, and prioritize the effort necessary to make it happen.

Communication—The Key Ingredient

If there is a single piece of advice that can help you deal with every type of intimacy problem that caregiving brings, it would surely be that you must talk about your feelings. It's important to share your feelings of frustration. Pretending that everything is okay is not healthy. The goal of expressing your feelings is that everyone will come to a better understanding of each other. Of course, the amount of expressiveness that works in each family will vary.

MEDICAL SITUATIONS: SOME OF WHAT YOU NEED TO KNOW

TIP SHEET #4

A Home Healthcare Primer

What Is Home Care?

Home care is the general term for a wide range of community-based services that can help support someone who is recuperating from an acute situation, such as a hip fracture, or services needed by persons with ongoing chronic conditions, such as stroke or cerebral palsy. The skills and duties of home care personnel vary, but all have one thing in common—they make it possible for care recipients to remain at home in a safe environment and in some cases have more independence than they did before. In the process, they also provide family care-givers with a chance to replenish their depleted physical and emotional reserves.

Home care personnel include:

- Registered nurses (RNs)—they provide skilled medical care, including giving medications, monitoring vital signs, dressing wounds, and teaching family caregivers how to use complicated equipment at home.
- Therapists—they work with patients to restore or main-tain their motor, speech, and cognitive skills.
- Home care aides—they provide personal services such as bathing, dressing, toileting, making meals, light cleaning, and transporting patients to the doctor.
- Companion/homemakers—they help with chores around the house but usually do not perform personal duties for the care recipient.

Getting Started with Home Care

If you are considering getting home care help to assist you with your caregiving responsibilities and/or to get some time for yourself, there are a number of things you need to consider, and also things you need to know.

- The first step is to make sure you and your loved one are comfortable with the idea of someone else taking on some of the tasks that you've been doing by yourself. There are many care recipients that are totally opposed to the idea, and some negotiations may need to occur before any plan can be put in place. It is important for all concerned to understand what is prompting the need for home care and the personal issues that lie beneath refusing to consider it. Getting beyond objections isn't necessarily easy and

you might need some guidance on how to go about it, perhaps from other family caregivers that have dealt with the
issue or from professionals who counsel family caregivers.

- Defining the tasks that need to be done by the home care
  worker will help you determine exactly what type of
  home care is most appropriate in your situation. Do you
  need a nurse to clean and bandage wounds and monitor
  equipment, a home care aide to help your loved one get
  showered and dressed, or a companion/homemaker to
  take care of some household duties?

- Once you know what type of assistance you need, and all
  parties agree that it is necessary or desirable, the inevitable questions about where to find home care services,
  how much they will cost, and whether any of the cost is
  covered by insurance or provided by government programs must be asked and answered. Some federally
  funded programs, insurance companies, and health maintenance organizations (HMOs) do provide for some home
  healthcare services, but the coverage provided may not fit
  your needs. To be sure whether you have any coverage at
  all, it is imperative that you review your insurance benefits.

- If you're like the majority of family caregivers, you need
  the most help with personal care tasks—the very type of
  care that is not typically covered by private health insurance programs or Medicare. So unless your loved one had
  the foresight and the funds to purchase long-term-care insurance prior to becoming ill, your access to home care
  will be limited by what you can afford. You may be able
  to get some help from state programs that take into account your ability to pay, and the age or extent of disability of your care recipient, but the sad reality is that the
  costs of home care services usually have to come out of
  your own pocket.

Choosing the Right Home Care

How do you find the right home care solution for your family, the one that provides the services you need at a price you can afford? There are several ways of tapping into the home care network. Here is a look at some of the most common ones and what you need to think about when considering them.

- Home Care Agencies are companies in the business of meeting home care needs. Not all home care agencies provide the same variety and level of service however, so make sure the agency you are considering can provide all the services you need. The issue isn't the size of the company but rather which one meets your criteria.
- If your care recipient is approved for skilled care that Medicare will pay for, it's vital that the agency be Medicare certified. This ensures that the agency has met federal minimum requirements. If your loved one only requires personal care or companion/homemaker care, Medicare certification need not be a factor in your decision. Some companies actually have two agencies that are legally separate but work together, one that is Medicare certified and one that is strictly private pay.
- Some agencies are accredited in addition to being certified. Well-known accrediting organizations are the National League for Nursing, the Joint Committee for Accreditation of Healthcare Organizations, and the National Foundation of Hospice and Home Care. This type of certification tells you that the agency conforms to national industry standards, and there is always comfort in knowing you are dealing with an organization that has proven its worth to its peers.
- What do home care services cost through an agency? Some agencies charge flat fees ranging from $100 to $120 per visit. Others have a minimum two or four-hour fee.

The actual hourly rate will vary depending on the services you require and the part of the country you live in, but don't be surprised to find rates ranging anywhere from $13 to $35 per hour.

Questions to Ask Any Agency You Are Thinking of Working With

- Is the agency certified for participation in Medicare and Medicaid programs (where applicable)?
- How long has the agency been serving the community?
- Is the agency accredited by the Joint Commission On Accreditation of Healthcare Organizations (JCAHO), Community Health Accreditation Program (CHAP), or another recognized accrediting body?
- Does the agency provide an initial assessment to determine if the patient would be appropriate for home care and what those services might be?
- Does the agency provide all of the services you need? Can it provide flexibility to meet the patient's changing health care needs?
- How does the agency choose and train its employees? Are background checks made? Does it protect its caregivers with written personnel policies, benefit packages, and malpractice insurance?
- Does the agency provide literature explaining its services, eligibility requirements, fees, and funding?
- Does the agency have arrangements in place for emergencies? Are the agency's caregivers available twenty-four hours a day, seven days a week? How quickly can they start service?
- Are references from former clients and doctors available?
- What types of programs does the company have in place to assure quality care is provided?
- Will the agency go to bat for you if your insurance com-

pany or Medicare fails to cover a claim you and the agency thought should be covered?

Privately Employed Home Caregivers

Instead of using a home care agency, you may wish to hire a home care worker on your own, especially if you are not looking for skilled medical care, but rather for someone to act as a companion or personal aide on a regular, long-term basis. In those situations, bypassing commercial agencies can often result in significant financial savings. You can start your search by putting the word out to friends and neighbors that may know of a home care worker. Also check with the nursing staff in your doctor's office, a hospital discharge planner, or community-based social service agencies for reliable candidates.

Things to Think About if You Plan to Hire Private Home Care Help

- You yourself must do substantial background checks to ensure that the employee has no record of criminal activity or abuse.
- You must be prepared to do all the paperwork necessary to comply with tax and insurance laws affecting employees.
- You may not get candidates with the same level of training and licensure as those who work for home care agencies.
- You do not have the guarantee of substitute help if your home caregiver is ill or on vacation.

Home Care Registries

A good middle ground between home care agencies and hiring help on your own is a home care registry. Registries are somewhat like employment agencies. They screen, interview, and reference-check workers they refer to clients so you don't have to, but just as with home care agencies, you need to ask a lot of questions to assure yourself that they can provide the right personnel to meet your needs. Because members of a registry are independent contractors, their services are available at prices that are usually lower than agencies.

Government In-home Aide Services

Many states and counties offer home care services to residents who are aged or disabled. Some even offer services to family caregivers. Applications for aid are evaluated by state social workers that rank a candidate's needs according to a number of objective criteria, including whether the care recipient lives alone and what activities he or she can perform. Care recipients who qualify are provided with home care aides who can give personal (not medical) care, do light cleaning, change linens, prepare meals, and transport or escort the patient to the doctor.

The aides are trained and licensed by the state. Fees are usually set on a sliding scale and can range anywhere from $1 to $20/hour depending on the care recipient's ability to pay. To find out what services your state offers, call your state Department of Human Resources or state Health Department. But be forewarned: These agencies are usually overwhelmed with applications and the waiting list can be long.

Hospice

If you are caring for a loved one with a terminal illness, hospice offers a number of services that can help. To qualify for in-home hospice care, you must have a doctor certify that your loved one is no longer seeking curative treatments and that he or she has "months rather than years to live." Depending on your situation, hospice will provide a social worker, a nurse who comes regularly to check medicines and vital signs, volunteers to sit with your loved one while you run errands or just get some rest, and home health aides who will bathe and clean the patient, tidy up the room, and fix a meal if necessary. Payment is usually through Medicare or private insurance. When you call your local hospice office, a home healthcare coordinator will work with you to arrive at the best combination of services for your situation.

TIP SHEET #5

When Your Loved One Is Hospitalized

Caregivers know all too well the feelings of helplessness that accompany their role of caring for a loved one with a chronic illness. When a hospitalization is involved, it is not uncommon to feel as though you have lost all control. There are steps you can take to ease the stress of a hospitalization and to ensure that you remain a part of the healthcare team should a hospital stay take place.

Most patients enter the hospital today as the result of a serious complication of a chronic illness or a life-threatening acute event. Because your loved one is likely to be seriously ill, there may be a great deal of uncertainty involved with his/her prognosis. Your loved one may experience a significant decline in function, and you may be forced to make crucial decisions without his/her input. By being proactive now, prior to any hospitalization, you will ensure that you and your loved one have a voice when it counts the most.

The Papers You Need

Having the proper legal documents in place is critical if you want to ensure that your loved one will receive the type of care they want and need. The following list outlines the basic documents we all should have.

- Durable Power of Attorney for Healthcare

  A durable power of attorney for healthcare, also known as a healthcare agent or proxy, is an individual you have appointed to make decisions about your medical care if you become unconscious or can no longer speak for yourself. A healthcare agent can be assigned as part of the advance directive form.

- Advance Medical Directive

  An advance directive informs your physician and family members what kind of care you wish to receive in the event that you can no longer make your own medical decisions.

- Living Will

  A living will is a type of advance directive that outlines what kind of medical treatment you want in certain situations. It only comes into effect if you are diagnosed with a terminal illness and have less than six months to live, or if you are in a persistent vegetative state. A living will does not, however, allow you to name someone to make decisions on your behalf.

- Do-Not-Resuscitate Order

  A do-not-resuscitate order (DNR) is a signed order directing that no cardiopulmonary resuscitative efforts (efforts to restart the heart after it has stopped) are to be undertaken in the event that your heart stops beating or you stop breathing. A DNR can be part of your advance directive. Does your loved one want resuscitation to occur regardless of circumstances? What are his/her feelings about ventilators and other life-sustaining equipment? If the decision is made that cardiopulmonary resuscitation is not what your loved one desires, than a DNR order must be written by your physician.

Advance directives, living wills, and durable power of attorney forms are all simple documents to complete and samples may be obtained through your local hospital, your attorney, or your state's attorney general's office. Your physician may also have copies of some of these documents. Signed copies should be given to your family physician. The documents must also be placed in the hospital chart each time your loved one is hospitalized.

Information You Need to Provide to Hospital Personnel

In addition to having the vital documents mentioned above, you can facilitate your loved one's transition to the hospital by providing the healthcare team with the following information:

- The patient's medical history, in writing.
- A list of the patient's allergies.
- A list of current medications and dosages.
- A list of all physicians and consultants who are caring for your loved one, along with phone numbers.

Providing this information immediately upon admission to the hospital can save crucial hours and improve communication. Often the hospitalization begins in the emergency room. The above information will ensure that, in the busy emergency room setting, your loved one's care is facilitated and physicians familiar with his/her case are involved from the start.

The Healthcare Team

As a family caregiver, you are a part of the health care team, which also includes the attending physician, the hospital nurses, and a hospital social worker or case manager. Each of these individuals, including you, has a role in the hospitalization. Stand up for your role on the team. The other members of the healthcare team need your input in order to evaluate, educate, diagnose, advise, and treat your loved one. Here are four things you should do upon arrival at the hospital.

- Find out the name of the attending physician of record for your loved one. This is the individual who will be coordinating the care throughout his or her hospital stay. This physician will be the primary doctor on the case. The attending physician will be in communication with the other consulting physicians and know their recommendations. Sometimes it is necessary to talk to a consultant about a specific issue, but often the attending physician can summarize the entire treatment plan. Make sure you understand and agree with that plan. Don't hesitate to continue asking questions until you feel comfortable with the answers. You may find it helpful to keep a running list of questions that you wish to discuss each time you see the physician.
- The first time you speak with the attending physician, make sure to find out the best way to get in touch with him or her. Who will initiate the phone contact? At what number can the physician be reached and what are the best times to call? Make sure the "face sheet" in your loved one's hospital chart contains your name and your correct phone numbers.
- Get to know the nurses who are caring for your loved one. They can answer your day-to-day questions and are an excellent source of information and support. Don't be afraid to ask the nurses about any new procedures or changes in your loved one's course of treatment. They are the natural starting point for questions, and will direct you to the attending physician when necessary. This will cut down on

any frustration you might feel at not being able to reach your attending physician every time you have a new issue to discuss. Realize that the change of shifts is a very busy time for the nurses, so find out when the shifts occur and try to hold your questions until the nurse coming on duty has received his or her report.

- As soon as you are able, speak to a hospital social worker or case manager, whose job it is to help you with any discharge planning issues. In a sense, the discharge process begins at the time of admission in terms of you finding out everything you need to know. This includes discussing what follow-up is necessary after you leave the hospital, who will be providing home healthcare, if necessary, what home health equipment you might need, and who will be paying for these additional expenses, including any special transportation services. Make sure you obtain the numbers of all home health companies providing goods and services and the names and numbers of companies that will deliver the equipment. A hospitalization may be the transition to a nursing home or hospice setting. The hospital social worker or case manager should help you make a smooth transition and can provide support for you, the caregiver, as well as for the patient.

Maintaining Some Control

Medicine is full of "lesser of the evils" choices, and at no time is this truer than when a chronically ill patient is hospitalized. The goal of hospitalization in these cases is often symptom management, with the understanding that the underlying problem cannot be fixed. The focus in the hospital will be on palliation and management rather than cure. It is important for you, as the primary caregiver, to keep this in mind, and to strive to understand the risks and benefits of any proposed course of treatment. It is also your role to make clear

to everyone on the healthcare team what your loved one's
wishes are regarding short-and long-term treatment. By being
more proactive in your communication, you will not only
simplify everyone's jobs, you will maintain some degree of
control. At no time is your role as caregiver more important
than when you speak on behalf of the person you love.

Information for Tip Sheet #5 was provided by Patricia L.
Tomsko, M.D., who is board certified in family practice, geri-
atrics, and hospice and palliative medicine, and by her assistant Sandy Padwo Rogers.

TIP SHEET #6

Choosing a Nursing Home: A Caregiver's Guide

It seems virtually no one wants to go to a nursing home, and
most caregivers do not want to institutionalize their loved
ones. But even though you may be committed to home care
and have no intention of using the services of a nursing home,
circumstances may arise that make institutionalizing your
care recipient a necessity, not a choice. It is possible that after
a stay in the hospital your care recipient may need a period of
specialized care of the sort you can't provide at home. Or you
yourself may become ill and need to find a nursing facility that
can care for your loved one while you recuperate. Perhaps your
care recipient's condition will progress to a point where you
can no longer provide the level of care needed. At that point,
intermediate or skilled nursing care may be required on a long
term or even permanent basis. If any of these things occur, you
will find yourself, perhaps very unexpectedly, in the position
of needing to evaluate and choose a nursing home.

A Decision with Heavy Emotional Components

Like so many issues in caregiving, the decisions surrounding this process involve very practical considerations overlaid

with an emotional component. Feelings of sadness, relief, guilt, and a sense of having failed may all be experienced when the time comes to put a loved one in a nursing home. As time goes on, and the raw emotions of the moment subside, one of the most important areas of comfort will be knowing that you have chosen the right home for your care recipient.

Types of Care

It is impossible to choose a nursing facility without first determining the type of care your loved one needs. Not only will that information assist you in finding a home that provides the proper level of care, it will also be a major factor in determining what, if any, government aid (Medicare or Medicaid) your care recipient will be eligible for.

The three most common types of care are personal care (often referred to as custodial care), intermediate, and skilled nursing. Custodial care means that residents need help with personal activities such as dressing, bathing, and eating. This type of care is essentially non-medical and is administered by aides rather than trained medical personnel.

Residents who need rehabilitative therapy and medications in addition to personal care are candidates for intermediate care. Intermediate care is delivered by licensed therapists and registered or licensed practical nurses.

When the level of disability is such that the resident is not able to care for him- or herself and may even be bedridden, skilled nursing care is needed. It is administered by licensed medical personnel on the orders of an attending physician.

Taking Stock: What Kind of Care Is Needed?

A good starting point for evaluating your care recipient's health status is the list of activities of daily living (ADLs), which include bathing, dressing, eating, going to the toilet, continence, mobility, and getting in or out of bed and other transferring situations. An additional list, the instrumental activities of daily living (IADLs), which include cooking, cleaning, shopping, taking medicine, and paying bills, can also help give you an overall picture of your loved one's abilities. And of course, consultation with the doctor, who will most likely have had considerable experience in nursing home placements, can prove invaluable.

Finances: What Can We Afford? What Do We Need to Know About Basic and Supplemental Costs?

Nursing homes are expensive—$50,000 per year on average, so your choices may well be dictated by what financial resources are available. First, it is important to realize that Medicare only covers very specific types or combinations of care. Personal care without other necessary prescribed care is never covered. Medicare covers only 100 days in a skilled nursing facility; the first twenty are fully paid but you must contribute a co-payment for the remaining eighty days. If your care recipient's stay is covered by Medicare, the facility you choose must be Medicare-approved.

Medicaid does cover nursing home costs but you must meet strict financial guidelines to qualify. If you think your loved one might be a candidate for Medicaid coverage, it is wise to contact an elder care attorney, or other professional who can help you work out the details and apply for Medicaid-eligible certification.

Make sure you understand the home's daily or monthly rate, which basic services are covered in this rate, which cost extra, what your payment plan will be, and whether a deposit is required.

Choosing the Nursing Home: What to Look For

Your initial screening should provide you with a list of facilities that offer the type of care needed, are geographically convenient, are within your price range, and have available beds. The next step is to arrange a personal inspection visit at the facility that looks most promising. Areas that you should inquire about (some of these can be handled over the phone to save time during your on-site visit) include:

- Services

  Does the home provide physical, occupational, or speech therapy, religious services, social activities, laundry service, television? Be sure to ask which of these are included in the monthly fee and which entail special charges. Surcharges can add several hundred dollars to your monthly bill, and you need to factor these costs into your financial assessment.

- Staff

  Find out how many registered nurses are on the staff, how often the doctor visits, how many staff are on duty during the day and on the night shift and what is the ratio of staff to patients, whether dental care is provided in-house, whether a pharmacist or other trained person maintains and reviews medication records on patients, how much turn-over there is among the staff, and what arrangements have been made for ambulance service.

- Accreditation

  If your care recipient qualifies (or may qualify in the future) for Medicare or Medicaid, make certain that the institution is certified by these programs. It should also be licensed by the state. Other accreditations, such as those from the Joint Commission of the Accreditation of Hospitals (JCAH) may provide further assurance, but the first two are absolute necessities.

  Examine the survey reports that are mandated for each nursing home by federal law. The state health department must inspect each facility to see that it meets certain minimum standards, then issues a deficiency report detailing problems found. This report should be displayed at the home. If it is not, ask to see it. If the facility can't seem to find the report while you are there, you will want to note that fact. However, don't be swayed solely by the number of deficiencies. A home that has numerous small, easily correctable deficiencies may be much more desirable than one which has fewer, but far more serious ones.

As You Tour the Facility, Consider These Areas

- Safety

  Are there sufficient smoke detectors, emergency exits, wheelchair ramps, call buttons, hand and guardrails in bathrooms and bedrooms?

- Livability

  Do the current residents look clean and cared for; are they engaged in varied activities, or are they simply sitting and staring? Are there opportunities to sit or recreate outdoors? Are physical restraints excessively used?

  Are the rooms of a decent size, with space for the residents' belongings? Are the rooms bright and cheerful? Can the residents decorate their rooms to some degree? Is there adequate privacy? Are the common rooms clean and welcoming or is there a pervasive, unpleasant odor? Does the staff treat residents respectfully and kindly? Does the staff radiate a generally pleasant and cheerful demeanor?

- Nutrition

  Is the food nutritious and appealing? Are fresh fruits and vegetables available? Are snacks served? Is the menu varied? Are special (low salt or low cholesterol) diets available? Does the staff feed those who can't feed themselves? Do the current residents say they like the food?

Tips from Those Who Have Been There

If you can afford it, try using a nursing home for short term stays to determine how well it meets your family's needs.

The nursing home decision is a very emotional and stressful one. Seek out counseling either during the decision-making process or immediately after.

If your care recipient is mentally fit and younger than typical nursing home residents, try to find an institution that is, if not geared to a younger population, at least a place where there is some interaction with people of a similar age and where activities are planned with younger people in mind. Check out the facility's bulletin board. It can give you a good idea of what activities are actually being offered.

Plan Ahead

As difficult as it is, if you know your care recipient may be a future candidate for a nursing home, do some of the research ahead of time, when you are not feeling stressed about a time limit. This can increase your chances of finding the best possible facility because when the time does come you may need to make a decision in just a few days.

The Intangible Component

You do need to have a list of practical considerations when you're looking at a nursing home, just as you do when you are considering any other type of housing decision. But the answers on a checklist aren't necessarily the whole story. Sometimes you find a place that's not as beautiful or as good on paper as some of the others, but you can just tell it has heart.

LEGAL AND FINANCIAL FACTS AND FIGURES

──────────◯ TIP SHEET #7 ◯──────────

Tax Tips for Family Caregivers

Information for this article was provided by Cecily Slater, CPA.

April 15 will probably never win any prizes as a favorite day for most Americans. As a caregiver, however, you may find that you are entitled to deductions or credits that can help take some of the sting out of the dreaded tax day. Tax rules change, so take these tips as a guide, but always check with a tax professional when you area getting ready to file.

Medical Expense Deductions—General Principles

For a deduction to qualify as a medical expense, you must have spent money to alleviate or prevent a physical or mental defect or illness. Common deductions include:

- Medical insurance premiums
- Prescription medicines
- Doctor's bills
- Hospital fees for services and/or room and board
- Travel to and from medical appointments.

You can deduct only medical and dental expenses that are in excess of 7.5% of your adjusted gross income (AGI). For example, if your AGI is $25,000 and your medical expenses add up to $2,000, you will be able to deduct only $125. That's the difference between the $2,000 you spent and $1,875, which is 7.5% of $25,000.

There's another catch—you can deduct only those amounts for which you have not been reimbursed by private insurance or Medicare. If you are in the upper tax brackets, some itemized deductions are phased out all together.

Special Expenses

You can claim the following special items as medical deductions:

- Oxygen and oxygen equipment
- Special schools or homes for the mentally or physically disabled (when recommended by a doctor)
- Artificial limbs
- False teeth
- Eyeglasses
- Wheelchairs and repairs
- Crutches
- Costs and care of guide dogs for aiding the disabled
- Braille books and magazines if they are more expensive than regular books and magazines
- Hearing aids and the batteries to operate them.

You can also deduct expenses for equipment or improvements you've made to your home for medical reasons, but the IRS will reduce these deductions by the amount such improvements increase the value of your home. Typical equipment and improvements added initially for medical reasons include:

- Ramps
- Widened doorways and hallways
- Grab bars in bathrooms
- Elevators, stair glides, etc.
- Air conditioning
- Accessible shower stalls

Unfortunately, health club dues and dancing or swimming lessons are not deductible, even if recommended by a doctor.

Nursing Home Care

Nursing home expenses, per se, are not deductible, but medical expenses incurred in a nursing home are. This includes the cost of meals and lodging while the patient is in the nursing home, so long as the main reason for being there is to get medical (not simply personal) care.

Nursing, Therapeutic, and/or Aide Services

Wages you pay for an attendant who provides nursing and/ or personal care services are deductible as medical expenses. These services include such nursing activities as giving medication and changing dressings, and typical personal care services such as bathing and grooming the patient.

If you provide room and board, these may also be deductible, but typical household services such as cooking and cleaning do not qualify as medical deductions.

For Whom Can You Claim Medical Deductions?

You can take medical expense deductions for yourself, your spouse, and your dependents. A person generally qualifies as a dependent for medical expense deductions if he or she meets all of the following criteria:

- Is related to you
- Lived with you for the entire year as member of your household
- Was a U.S. citizen or resident, or a resident of Canada or Mexico, for at least part of the calendar year for which you are filing taxes
- You provided over half of that person's total support for the calendar year. If you and someone else are providing more than half a dependent's support, but no one alone provides more than half, you can use what's called a "multiple support agreement" to claim the dependent, but only one of the parties to the multiple support agree-

ment can claim medical expenses for the dependent person. In the case of divorced parents, however, the child is considered a dependent of both parents for the medical expense deduction.

Where to Get Help

Tax law is confusing at best. If you want some additional information, here are ways to get it:

- The Internal Revenue Service offers a number of publications that can help you understand the deductions and tax credits you may be entitled to. Some of the most helpful include:
  - Your Federal Income Tax—Publication 17
  - Medical and Dental Expenses—Publication 502
  - Credit for the Elderly or Disabled—Publication 554
  - Tax Rules for Children and Dependents—Publication 929

  To order these publications, call 1-800-TAX-FORM.
- The IRS will also answer taxpayer questions if they are not too complicated or controversial. But you must realize, while the IRS will try to guide you in finding the answers you need, it does not offer tax advice. To find the Taxpayer Service Number for your area, check the local phone book under the IRS listings.
- There is only one place to go for individual tax advice, and that is to a tax professional. If you are confused about what deductions or credits may apply to you, or if you need help preparing your return, you may find it beneficial to consult someone who specializes in this area. There are a number of tax services available, and you can find their numbers in the phone book, but the best refer-

ence may well be word of mouth. Talk to people you know and respect and ask them for a referral.

⟐ TIP SHEET #8 ⟐

What If I Die? A Planning Guide for Caregivers

Information for this article was reviewed by David Mosell, Attorney at Law and originally compiled by Ronald Landsman, also an attorney. Mr. Mosell specializes in estate planning, Mr. Landsman in elder law.

What if I die? This is not a question most caregivers think about, unless they are ill themselves or are caring for someone much younger than they are. But it is wise to remember that all of us can get hit by the proverbial bus. Caregivers, more than most people, need to ask the question, "What if I die?" And having asked it, they need to make plans—just in case. Here are some things that you as a caregiver need to consider regarding care for your loved one in the event of your own premature death.

There are three fundamental questions to consider:

1. What level of care do you provide, and who would fill your shoes if you died?
2. Who should receive your assets, and how do you want them used?
3. How can the income that you bring in now (either because you are working or because you receive social security benefits, a pension, etc.) be at least partially replaced?

A will provides the answers to the first two questions. Life insurance and retirement survivor benefits can help provide answers to the third.

What Your Will Should Contain

A typical will for a married person says "everything to my spouse, but if he or she predeceases me, then everything to my children." Such sweetheart wills are ideal for slightly older families in which the children are grown and healthy, and the parent's estate does not exceed the current estate tax limit. But for caregivers, sweetheart wills are a disaster waiting to happen.

Naming a Guardian

Your will should not be the same as that of a non-caregiver. For one thing, it should address the issue of guardianship of your loved one. If you are the guardian now, whom do you want to replace you? And if that person were to die as well, whom do you want to name as a backup?

These are difficult questions to answer and can take a long time to resolve. Most people choose a family member, but not always. You need to name the person that you think will make the best decisions for your loved one, regardless of whether that person is a family member.

Disbursing Your Property

If the person you are caring for is not mentally competent, is a minor, or could benefit from Medicaid coverage (this includes most unemployed people and many disabled persons as well), then you shouldn't leave money to him or her outright because it will be put into a conservatorship. The money will be managed, but not necessarily by someone you want. In addition, if you leave the money outright, he or she will lose Medicaid benefits, at least temporarily.

Generally speaking, money should be put in a discretionary trust. This will allow the trustee(s) you have named to use his or her own discretion (hence its name) about how funds should be used to provide the best care and most comfortable life for your loved one. If the trust stipulates the funds can be used for support and maintenance, your loved one will not be able to benefit from Medicaid at all until all of the monies in the trust are exhausted. This is particularly true for people who have fallen outside of the traditional insurance network, such as an unemployed 25-year-old or an adult who has left the work-force because of medical issues.

Insurance Planning

The purpose of life insurance for caregivers is twofold:

1. To replace the income stream that will be lost at your death, whether it be actual salary or pension benefits of some kind;

2. To provide an asset that will generate the income needed to pay for the services you are currently providing free of charge.

All assets that name a beneficiary—insurance, an IRA, or a pension plan with survivor benefits—should be coordinated with your will. You will need to name a beneficiary to receive these assets after your death. Unless the person for whom you are caring is fully competent, you should not name him or her, but rather the trustee of the trust that you have established in your will.

If all of this sounds very technical, that's because it is. You may be able to relate to it better by reading the following case studies. One deals with an adult child of an aged parent, another with a spousal caregiving relationship, and the third with parents of a child with a disability.

If You're Caring for Mom

Jack Porter is 50 years old. He has no siblings. He is married to Kate, and they have two children: Anne, 20 and Chris, 16.

Anne is a sophomore in college. Chris wants to become a doctor. Jack's mom, Mrs. Porter, has Parkinson's disease. At the moment, she is quite competent, and she has named Jack to be her guardian if and when she becomes incompetent. Jack, in his own will, should name a backup guardian just in case he dies before his mom. Mrs. Porter should do the same. If Kate and Mrs. Porter have agreed that when Jack dies, Kate will become Mrs. Porter's caregiver and guardian, Jack doesn't have to make special provisions in his will. However, if he wants to ensure that there are assets specifically set aside for his mother's care, he needs to make a separate provision in his will for that purpose. In addition, he must have assets in his own name, as opposed to in both his and Kate's names, to fund the bequest. If he doesn't, then Kate would automatically inherit everything.

As a member of the sandwich generation, Jack has to balance the needs of his mother with the needs of his children, and allocate his resources accordingly. The problem is that he doesn't know whether his children will still be in school when he dies or already out on their own. One option is to set up a discretionary trust (remember, that's better than a support and maintenance trust), that comes into play only if both he and Kate predecease Mrs. Porter. Jack can name Mrs. Porter, Anne, and Chris as beneficiaries and let the trustee determine how to disburse the funds based on each one's needs at the time.

When Your Spouse Is Disabled or Ill

Leslie's husband, Aaron, is paraplegic. Mentally he is fine, but physically he requires assistance with the activities of daily living. Their children are grown, and although caring and supportive, all have families of their own and live in distant states. To plan for future eventualities, Aaron should name someone to act for him in both financial and healthcare matters in the event he does become incompetent. Presumably he will choose Leslie, but it could even be one of his children, despite the fact that they live far away.

Beyond that, unless Aaron and Leslie have significant assets to protect, they need not make special arrangements. If they do have significant assets, Leslie may want to consider writing a will with a discretionary trust. It would be funded in the event of her death, either because all assets are in her name, or because they are in a revocable trust that "pours over" into the will upon her death. (I know this sounds very complicated, but it is really fairly straightforward, and your attorney, if he or she specializes in estate planning for incapacity, will be able to give you a further explanation.) Leslie may also want to consider buying additional life insurance because Aaron may need the money to pay for his own care when she is gone. The money would go into the trust upon her death.

When Your Child Is Truly Dependent

John and Paula Watkins are in their thirties. They have two children. Thomas is one year old and is a healthy baby. Melanie is six and has cerebral palsy. John and Paula's parents are still alive, but live far away. Paula has two sisters who live nearby. Paula is a fulltime homemaker and caregiver. John is a policeman.

Obviously, if either John or Paula die the other would continue as the guardian of their children. They do need, however, to address the issue of who would take over if they both die. They will need to decide whether one person should be named to care for both children or, because Melanie needs so much more care, whether two separate guardians should be named. These are not easy decisions to make and require much thought and discussion with other family members. In addition, they need to take into account the fact that now John is providing all of the family income. With proper insurance coverage and survivor benefits from the police force, his income can be replaced. If Paula dies, however, John's income needs to increase because Paula has been providing services free of charge. John and Paula will need to figure out what it would cost to hire a fulltime housekeeper to replace Paula, and possibly other help as well. This calculation needs to be part of the determination of how much insurance there should be on Paula's life. Because she is relatively young and quite healthy she should be able to get a considerable amount of term insurance for a relatively low rate.

Another thing that John and Paula need to think about is how funds should be distributed for the care of Thomas and Melanie because their needs are so different. One approach is for both John and Paula to leave all of their assets to each other. In the event they both die, funds should go into a discretionary trust. (This is something that all parents with dependent children should do, regardless of whether the kids are healthy or ill.) To some extent, if they have enough life insurance, how the funds should be allocated can be left to the trustee. John and Paula are perhaps in the most difficult situation of the families in these scenarios because the dependent person in their family is most likely to live for a very long time after their demise. This is all the more reason why they need to plan carefully now, when they have options.

In Conclusion

Nobody likes to think about death, especially his or her own. But death comes to us all, sometimes unexpectedly, and because of that, death planning now can save a great deal of heartache and pain for your dependent loved one who survives. Making plans for his or her care after you are gone is one of the most caring things you can do now.

APPENDIX C

Written Testimony
of
Suzanne Mintz, President/Co-founder
National Family Caregivers Association
Presented to
U.S. Senate Subcommittee on Oversight of Government Management,
Restructuring and the District of Columbia
On July 24, 2001
Hearing Title: Who Cares for the Caregivers?: The Role of Health
Insurance in Promoting Quality Care for Seniors, Children and
Individuals with Disabilities

Mr. Chairman, members of the Committee, thank you for this opportunity. My name is Suzanne Mintz, and I am the President and Co-founder of the National Family Caregivers Association (NFCA). NFCA exists to educate, support, and empower family caregivers and speak out publicly for meeting caregivers' needs. We reach across the boundaries of differing diagnoses, different relationships, and different life stages to address the common concerns of all family caregivers.

Our members care for spouses, children, aging parents, siblings, friends, and others. Half are caring for seniors 66 or older, and most are "heavy duty" caregivers, meaning they are providing extensive hands-on care on a daily basis, helping loved ones, dress, bath, toilet, etc. For three fifths of these caregivers, caregiving is the equivalent of more than a full-time job.

I have been asked to speak to you about the role of family caregivers in our society, the impact of being a family caregiver, and the need for family caregivers to have health insurance. Family caregivers are defined as those individuals who provide uncompensated care to a family member or friend who needs care because he or she is chronically ill, disabled, or elderly.

Although the term *family caregiver* is now understood by many, I do not believe that the role family caregivers play in society is thoroughly appreciated. Family caregivers are literally underpinning the American healthcare system.

The vast majority of care provided to chronically ill or disabled individuals is provided by family members. Approximately three-quarters of non-institutionalized adults ages 18–64 receive all of their care from family caregivers.[i] When we look at the 65+ population, approximately two thirds of those needing care receive it solely from family.[ii] More than 50 million people provide some level of care to a loved one.[iii]

The conservative market value of services provided by family caregivers to adults was estimated in 1997 to be $196 billion dollars.[iv] And the number of family caregivers in America is growing as the population ages, as medical science continues to extend the lives of those with chronic illness, and as healthcare containment policies send people home from hospitals sooner and in need of more care than ever before.

As former first lady Rosalynn Carter has said in her book, *Helping Yourself Help Others:*

> There are only four kinds of people in the world—
> those who are currently caregivers,
> those who have been caregivers,
> those who will be caregivers, and
> those who will need caregivers.

Caregiving is often a continuum. For many it begins by providing a small amount of assistance to an aging parent or spouse with a degenerative disease and then over time becomes a 24/7 experience. For others, intensive caregiving begins very sud-

denly, as when a baby is born severely ill, or when a loved one
is in a terrible car accident or has a massive stroke.

> *I am a 35-year-old mother of a 5-year-old severely disabled
> daughter, Kaylee, who suffers from a rare genetic disorder
> called Camptomelic Dysplasia. . . . Kaylee requires 24 hour
> medical care.*

The typical family caregiver provides an average of between
18–20 hours of care each week to a loved one 50 and older, virtually the equivalent of a half-time job. Caregivers in over four
million households provide at least 40 hours of care a week.[v]
In a recent survey of New York City caregivers providing care
to a loved one of any age, 40% were providing 20 hours of care
a week or more.[vi] Over half of Alzheimer's caregivers, who are
seniors themselves, provide 41 or more hours of care per
week.[vii]

The surveys of family caregivers show that the number of
caregiving hours has a direct correlation with the amount and
type of help the care recipient requires. For instance, those
helping a loved one who has a degenerative disease such as
multiple sclerosis, ALS, or Parkinson's, and help with a combination of several activities of daily living, such as bathing,
dressing, transferring, and toileting, are known to provide
more hours of care than those who are helping someone solely
with money management, food preparation, or transportation.

> *We get up at 5 a.m. I get grandmother washed, dressed and put
> her in her wheelchair. While she is brushing her teeth, I get my
> 4-year-old and 18-month-old ready for the day. At 7:15,
> grandma gets on the Easter Seals bus to go to adult day care.
> My kids go to a babysitter, and then I work at a hospice all day.
> Depending on the day, I usually get home around 3:30 p.m. If I
> have a chance, I take a shower. If I don't, I start making dinner.
> Grandma gets home around 4:00. My kids get home around
> 4:15. We have dinner and then around 7:00 I get grandma
> ready for bed. Then I hit the bed . . . heavy . . . I figure that my*

*grandmother changed my diapers when I was a kid, and now
it's time for me to change hers.*

The physical and emotional impact of intensive family caregiving has been well documented.[viii] As you would imagine,
there is a correlation between the numbers of hours of caregiving, the extent of physical assistance provided and the actual impact of the caregiving experience. These caregivers are
known to suffer more depression and other stress-related ail-
ments than the general population. In an NFCA member survey, 61% of caregivers reported depression, 51% sleeplessness,
41% back problems.[ix] One study of elderly spousal caregivers
showed that 63% of those experiencing stress had a higher
mortality rate than those not stressed or in a caregiving situation.[x]

*I am just stressed out. I have come to a point where I am just
really worried all the time. Sometimes I know I'm here, but
it's hard to believe it. It seems like I'm in a dream world or
something. I'm exhausted.*

The impact of caregiving is not only physical or mental. It can
also be social and financial. Caregivers report feelings of isolation, a distance from "normal" life, and a feeling that no one
else could understand what they are going through.

*His condition caught us completely off guard, especially since
we consider ourselves too young to have this seriously out of
control health problem. I have so many newly discovered feelings: mostly, I feel a sense of tremendous loneliness and occa-
sionally depression for the lifestyle I miss from before his illness and guilt about feeling the way I do.*

Caregiving is expensive. Families in which one person has a
disability and needs help with daily living activities spend two
and one half times more out of pocket on medical expenses
than families without a disabled person.[xi] Thirty-five percent
of the general population has an income of less than $30,000.

Among family caregivers that percentage rises to 43%.[xii] Caregiving literally extracts a price from caregiving families.

The majority of family caregivers are employed, nearly 64%,[xiii] but over a third have reduced their work hours or taken time off because of caregiving responsibilities.[xiv] Six percent of those caring for the 50+ population have left the workforce because of their caregiver responsibilities.[xv] Forty-two percent of young parents of special needs children lack basic workplace supports, such as paid sick leave and vacation time.[xvi] Adding to the problem, family caregivers that leave the workforce not only lose their paycheck, they lose the future benefit of the additional social security credits they would have earned.

Although I am not familiar with any studies that document how many caregivers have lost their group health insurance because they have left the workforce, anecdotal information from NFCA members suggest that for some caregivers that is the case.

"I had to give up both work and health insurance for a period of 6 years due to caregiving responsibilities."

"My husband's job 'disappeared' after his stroke in 1998 and with it our medical coverage."

"I lost my business, health insurance and most of my savings due to the stress of caring for somebody as ill as my wife Beverly. Also I have two young children to care for and raise."

"I quit work to care for my husband and paid an exorbitant amount for COBRA insurance for both of us. When that ran out, I had to get an individual policy (which he was not eligible for) and pay for it myself."

"I have been caregiver for my mother and aunt, both in their 80's, since 1991. I had to quit my job last year when my mother had another heart attack. I lost health, dental, vision, and disability insurance, plus pension and deferred compensation. I am presently retaining my health insurance through

COBRA, but it costs me $304 per month and it will run out on 1/1/02."

Not surprisingly, recent research on the impact that not having health insurance has on individuals and families documents that those without health insurance are twice as likely as the insured to have difficulty obtaining care for themselves and their families. For instance uninsured persons with chronic back problems (often an issue for family caregivers) are three times as likely as insured persons not to have access to a regular source of care.[xvii]

It is clear that family caregivers are making a tremendous contribution, not only to their individual loved ones, but to American society as a whole, and some of them are doing so at a huge physical, emotional, and financial cost. The work that family caregivers do, the uncompensated work of caregiving that is done with feelings of love and out of a sense of duty, needs to be valued and supported in direct and meaningful ways.

Without family caregivers our current healthcare system could not function. The length of hospital stays, the need for institutionalization and professional home care services would expand significantly. Therefore, it is in the government's interest to help ensure the health of family caregivers by providing free health insurance to those caregivers who need it. If a family caregiver gets sick, or dies, who then will care for their loved one? It is less costly, more humane, and better policy to protect the health of family caregivers while we can. Providing them with quality health insurance is one of the ways to do that.

Endnotes

[i] Tilly, Goldenson, Kasten, O'Shaughnessy, Kelly and Sidor, *Long-Term Care Chart Book: Persons Served, Payors and Spending*, The Urban Institute and Congressional Research Service, 2000.

[ii] Assistant Secretary for Planning and Evaluation, Administration on Aging, *Informal Caregiving: Compassion in Action*, 1998.

[iii] Idem, *Informal Caregiving: Compassion in Action* and National Family Caregivers Association, *Survey 2000*, unpublished.

[iv] Arno, Levine, Memmott, *The Economic Value of Informal Caregiving*, *Health Affairs* 18/2, 1999. (This has recently been updated.)

[v] As above, *Informal Caregiving: Compassion in Action* and National Alliance for Caregiving (NAC)/AARP, *Family Caregiving in the U.S.* 1997.

[vi] Levine, Kuerbis, Gould, Navaie-Walise, Feldman, Donelan, *A Survey of Family Caregivers in New York City: Findings and Implications for the Health Care System*, A Special Report from the United Hospital Fund and Visiting Nurse Service of New York, 2001.

[vii] Alzheimer's Association/National Alliance for Caregiving, *Who Cares? Families Caring for Persons with Alzheimer's Disease*, 1998.

[viii] Shulz, Visintainer, Williamson, "Psychiatric and Physical Morbidity Effects of Caregiving", *Journal of Gerontology*, 1990, Vol. 45.

[ix] National Family Caregivers Association, *Caregiving Across the Life Cycle*, 1998.

[x] Schultz, Beach, "Caregiving as a Risk Factor for Mortality: The Caregiver Health Effects Study", Journal of the American Medical Association, December 15, 1999, Vol. 282, No. 23.

[xi] Altman, Cooper, Cunningham, *The Case of Disability in the Family: Impact on Health Care Utilization and Expenditures for Non-disabled Members*, Millbank Quarterly, 77, 1999.

[xii] As above, NFCA *Survey 2000*.

[xiii] As above, *Informal Caregiving: Compassion in Action* and *Family Caregiving in the U.S.*

[xiv] Bond, Gainsky, Swanberg, *National Study of the Changing Workforce*, 1998.

[xv] As above, *Family Caregiving in the U.S.*

[xvi] Heymann, *The Widening Gap: Why America's Working Families are in Jeopardy and What Can be Done About It*, January 2000.

[xvii] Families USA, *Getting Less Care: The Uninsured with Chronic Health Conditions*, 2001.

Selected Chapter Bibliography

Only books, articles, and studies specifically mentioned by name in the text are included here. Many more sources were used in researching information for this book.

Introduction

Levine Carol ed., *Always on Call, When Illness Turns Families into Caregivers.* New York: United Hospital Fund (2000) 2.

Chapter 1

Styron, William., *Darkness Visible: A Memoir of Madness.* New York: Random House, (1990) 50.

Chapter 2

Cassidy Wiggins, Rita. *Shedding Light: Poems About Living With Alzheimer's.* St. Helena: Ten Press, (2000) 13.
Dickinson, Peter. *Some Death before Dying.* New York: Mysterious Press, Warner Books, (1999) 21.
Mace, Nancy L., M.A., and Rabins, Peter V., M.D., M. P.H. *36 Hour Day, A Family Guide to Caring for Someone with Alzheimer's Disease, Related Dementing Illnesses, and Memory Loss in Later Life.* Baltimore: Johns Hopkins Press, 1999.

Chapter 4

Bly, Robert, *Morning Poems*, New York: Harper Collins (1997).
Clooney, Eleanor, *Death in Slow Motion: My Mother's Descent into Alzheimer's.* To be published in January 2003.
Harper's Magazine Vol 303 # 19817 (2001): 43–58.
Jivanjee, Pauline PhD, Simpson, Jennifer PhD, "Respite Care for Children with Serious Emotional Disorders and Their Families: A

Way to Enrich Family Live." *Focal Point*, Regional Research Institute for Human Services Portland State University Vol 15 No 2 (2001).

Kiecolt-Glaser JK et al "Slowing of Wound Healing by Psychological Stress" *Lancet* Vol 346 (1995) 1194–1196.

Levine Carol ed., *Always on Call, When Illness Turns Families into Caregivers*. New York: United Hospital Fund (2000) 93–95.

Mittleman MS, et al. "A Family Intervention to Delay Nursing Home Placement of Patients with Alzheimer's Disease: A Randomized Controlled Trial" *Journal of the American Medical Association* Vol 276 (1996): 1725–1731.

National Family Caregivers Association, *Survey of Self-Identified Family Caregivers*, 2001.

Schulz, Richard PhD, "Caregiving as a Risk Factor for Mortality, The Caregiver Health Effects Study." *Journal of the American Medical Association* Vol 282 No 23 (1999): 2215–2219.

Chapter 5

National Alliance for Caregiving and American Association of Retired Persons, *Family Caregiving in the U.S.*: Findings from a National Survey, 1997.

Chapter 6

Lazaroff, Alan MD. Testimony "Cash Crunch: The Financial Challenge of LTC" Washington: Senate Special Committee on Aging (March 9, 1998).

Levine, Carol. *Rough Crossings: Family Caregivers' Odysseys through the Health Care System*. New York: United Hospital Fund (1998) 9, 11–13.

Mintz, Suzanne. Testimony "Who Cares for the Caregivers: The Role of Health Insurance in Promoting Quality Care for Seniors, Children, and Individuals with Disabilities" Washington: Senate Subcommittee on Oversight of Government Management Restructuring and the District of Columbia (July 24, 2001).

Shellenbarger Sue "Work & Family" *Wall Street Journal*, 13 September, 2000.

BIOGRAPHY FOR SUZANNE GEFFEN MINTZ, PRESIDENT AND CO-FOUNDER, NATIONAL FAMILY CAREGIVERS ASSOCIATION

Suzanne Mintz is a family caregiver for her husband (Steven) who was diagnosed with Multiple Sclerosis in 1974. In 1993, she, along with fellow caregiver Cindy Fowler, co-founded NFCA based on the belief that family caregivers were sorely in need of recognition, support, education, and advocacy. She has been its prime mover ever since.

One of the first to champion the now widely held belief that caregiving is a lifespan issue that should be treated as such rather than dealt with in silos of age, relationship, and diagnoses, Ms. Mintz soon became recognized as a far-sighted and responsible spokesperson for family caregivers, as attested to by her appearances before Congress, her participation in the crafting of national legislation, and her often sited remarks in major media outlets. Many of her efforts are focused on empowering other caregivers to speak up on behalf of their loved ones and themselves.

Suzanne is the author of the widely respected and distributed NFCA series of self-empowerment "action-oriented" educational pamphlets for family caregivers; a quarterly column for family caregivers in *Paraplegic News; The Resourceful Caregiver: Helping Family Caregivers Help Themselves;* and *Love, Honor, & Value: A Family Caregiver Speaks Out About the Choices and Challenges of Caregiving* (Sept 2002).

NFCA was established in 1993 to educate, support, empower, and advocate for the millions of Americans who care for their ill, aged, or disabled loved ones. NFCA reaches across the boundaries of different diagnoses, different relationships, and different life stages to address the common needs and concerns of all family caregivers. It is the only place that all caregivers can call "home."